# Communicate with Me – Access your online resources

*Communicate with Me* is accompanied by a number of printable online materials, designed to ensure this resource best supports your professional needs.

Activate your resources in three simple steps:

- Go to www.speechmark.net then create account / login

- Once registered, go to My Resources, where you'll be asked to enter the below activation code

- Once activated, all online resources that accompany *Communicate with Me* will appear in the My Resources section of your account – every time you log in

ACTIVATION CODE* –  **ujedbbeljt**                  Id:77

*Note, activation codes may be used on a one time only basis

A number of new Speechmark titles are accompanied by supporting materials, accessible online. Each time you purchase one, enter your unique activation code (typically found on the inside front cover of the resource) and enjoy access to My Resources – your very own online library of printable, practical resources that may be accessed again and again.

# Communicate *with* Me

## A Resource to Enable Effective Communication and Involvement with People Who Have a Learning Disability

Martin Goodwin, Jennie Miller and Cath Edwards

Foreword by Dr Nicola Grove

*Consultant in Communication and Narrative*
*Honorary Senior Lecturer, Tizard Centre*
*Founder of OpenStoryTellers (www.openstorytellers.org.uk)*

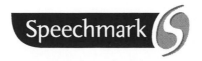

First published in 2015 by
Speechmark Publishing Ltd,
2nd Floor, 5 Thomas More Square, London E1W 1YW, UK
Tel: +44 (0)845 034 4610; Fax: +44 (0)845 034 4649
**www.speechmark.net**

Design and artwork by Moo Creative (Luton)

**002-5995**/Printed in the United Kingdom by CMP (uk) Ltd

British Library Cataloguing in Publication Data
A catalogue record for this book is available from the British Library

ISBN 978 191022 768 8

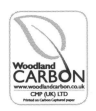

# Contents

# Contents

# Foreword

This splendid book is something we have needed for many years - forty in my case, since the day I emerged as a new and very nervous speech and language therapist to take up my posts in a special school and an adult day centre. If we can get communication partnerships right for those we support, so much else falls into place and works well. But language and communication are hugely complex areas, and it's not surprising that our efforts often end in breakdowns and misunderstandings.

Three of our most experienced practitioners in the field of learning/intellectual disabilities have managed to produce a guide that is theoretically sound, easy to read and highly practical in its approach. As a reader, you find you are easily absorbing a wealth of information because of the way that abstract ideas are followed by case studies – where you will recognise the children and adults who are part of your life – questions and reflections that lead you to understand puzzling behaviour in the light of how you yourself respond to the challenges they set, and examples of good practice that will inspire you because they are so eminently achievable.

I learned so much from reading it through – at last I can grasp the Mental Capacity Act! I can summarise the implications of the medical and social models of disability! It is wide ranging – moving from the person at the centre to the service and civic environments in which they function; and addressing so many of the everyday problems that come up time and time again: managing change, why training so often fails to result in effective implementation; decision making, and guidance on when and how to seek consultation. The website which backs up the resource means that there is an immediate interface and support available.

The first section of the resource provides the background information that must inform the way we view communication. It has long been recognised that communication is a multidimensional process, which encompasses not only the resources of the individual with a disability, but the values, attitudes and skills of interactive partners, the environment and the cultural context which determines both expectations and opportunities for growth and participation. *Communicate with Me* helps the reader to grasp this complex model, through its systematic approach. Framing the whole resource in the context of human rights and associated legislation emphasises for the reader that the people they work with are first and foremost fellow citizens. The discussion of models of disability allows due weight to be given to the significant challenges posed by impairments as well as social barriers, providing a balanced perspective.

Looking at individuals, it's impressive that the authors have managed to reference not only the obvious problems affecting communication but some of the subtle associated difficulties that can be masked in the way that a person behaves – attention, visual perception and acuity, literacy, memory and processing. The development of communication is explained clearly and with excellent practical examples, and clarifying the vital distinction between understanding and expression, and the value of adopting the philosophy of Total Communication. The crucial stage of intentionality in preverbal communication is given its due significance. I can remember trying to clarify for a support worker that when a lady with profound disabilities banged her tray continuously, this did not necessarily mean that she was making demands; how much easier my task would have been if I could have shown her this section! Practical suggestions of how to support people to communicate effectively at each stage are provided.

The second section of the book covers specific approaches and toolkits, once again within an overarching perspective of values, rights and responsibilities. There are so many imaginative and appealing ideas here that services can adopt, which will stimulate not only the people they support but their staff as well. I am longing to find someone who wants to decorate their room so I can create wallpaper collages with them (whether or not they have a learning disability); and I am going off to create an independence board to have in the car so I can change a tyre with confidence the next time I get a puncture.

In the third section, the authors move to looking at ways that services can promote genuine active involvement in society by people with learning disability: creating opportunities, providing accessible information, making choices, and using creative approaches including story, art and music.

Finally, services are invited to consider structures and systems that support communication. This is absolutely critical – as all speech and language therapists know, it is simply not possible to effectively develop the potential of people with learning disabilities unless the relevant structures are in place. I learned this early in my career when researching the use of signing in schools. There were many committed teachers and classroom assistants who used signs well within their classrooms – but the only schools where we saw signing between the pupils and signing outside instructional settings were the two schools where the senior management team had adopted signing as a policy and ensured that proper regular training was provided. Without this, a child could have good sign input one year, but move to a class where the teacher's view was "I'm not good with my hands" – and all the learning of the last 12 months could be undone. The quality assurance tools, which are online, help to bring all of this together so that the child or adult with a learning disability can receive a coordinated response to being communicated with.

The publication of this resource is timely. Services are shrinking and specialist support is contracting. People with learning disabilities need informed, committed and skillful partners in their struggle to take their rightful place in society – and this accessible, interactive and comprehensive guide will prove an invaluable support to everyone who has the privilege and the challenge of sharing their lives and work with people who have difficulties in communication.

**Nicola Grove**
www.drnicolagrove.com
*July 2015*

# Acknowledgements

The authors would like to dedicate this book to Penny Lacey. Dr Penny Lacey (1948–2015) was a senior lecturer in Severe and Profound Learning Disability at the University of Birmingham. Penny was an inspirational thinker and practitioner who was committed to supporting the development of approaches that improve the quality of life of people with learning disabilities. We will greatly miss Penny's dedication to her work, humour, compassion and insight.

The authors would like to thank Sarah Rooney (Retired Lecturer for University of Manchester), Ruth Miller (Speech and Language Therapist), Dr Penny Lacey (who was a senior lecturer at the University of Birmingham) and Dr Nicola Grove (Teacher and Speech and Language Therapist) for their support in reviewing the book and materials. Their contributions have been extremely valuable and we have been inspired by their practice in working with people with a learning disability and commitment to supporting development within the field. We would also like to thank Gillian Miller for reviewing early drafts of the book.

We would like to thank Sarah Ray for her illustrations (www.sarahray.com) and the following organisations for allowing us to include their images: Inspired Services, Widget Software and Mayer-Johnson LLC.

We would like to thank our publishers at Speechmark, who share our ambition in supporting individuals, settings and services to achieve effective communication with people with a learning disability.

Lastly, we would also like to thank the children, young people and adults with learning disabilities and parents who were part of the advisory group and projects for helping us to develop ideas for the book and quality assurance materials.

## From Martin

I would like to thank: my friends and family for their continued support; the people with whom I have collaborated to write this book, Jennie and Cath, for their dedicated support and passion; the professionals and academics who have inspired me to write this book; but, most of all, I would like to thank the children, young people and adults with learning disabilities from whom I continue to learn the most.

## From Jennie

I would like to thank all of the people who have inspired and influenced my work practice over the years – and who have motivated me to become a better practitioner myself so that I can make more of a difference in other people's lives and guide others to do the same. I especially thank anyone whose experiences I have captured as examples in this publication. I would like to thank Martin and Cath for our shared realisation of the vision Martin and I had for this publication one sunny day, walking through London seven years ago, and all the hours we have invested in between!

## From Cath

I would like to thank: those close to me for their support and care; Martin and Jennie for the many hours of hard work needed to put their considerable knowledge into this publication; the many talented and dedicated professionals, especially speech therapists, physiotherapists, psychologists and occupational therapists who have taught me so much and whose wisdom is reflected in these pages. And, last but far from least, the many children and adults with whom I have had the privilege of working over the years who showed such effort, commitment and ingenuity in doing their utmost to communicate with me.

## And finally ...

The journey of writing and developing *Communicate with Me* has been inspired and informed by challenges and good practice that some individuals, practitioners, settings and services have experienced with developing effective communication and involvement. *Communicate with Me* aims to make effective communication and involvement of people a reality so that people with learning disabilities have an improved quality of life. We hope that you join us on that journey by reflectively engaging with the book, keeping in touch and signing up to the Quality Assurance Schemes.

# Introduction to *Communicate with Me*

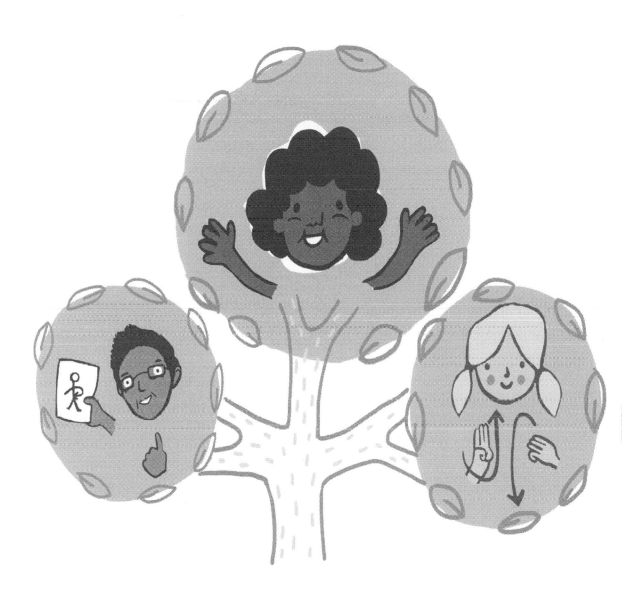

### *Communicate with Me* mission statement

*Communicate with Me* was written in response to a need to improve how the services for people with learning disabilities communicate with, and involve, the people they support. It was written as a resource to support work practice and a quality assurance tool to support services to integrate these practices into service culture. Communication is integral to delivering a quality service for people with a learning disability and effective communication enhances the quality of that support.

*Communicate with Me* is a resource that provides guidance to anyone who supports someone with a learning disability, whether they are a paid practitioner (employed by a service or directly by an individual), a family member, an advocate or another member of that person's community. This resource refers to these people as 'communication partners', which reflects the importance of equality in our relationships with people with learning disabilities.
The authors' vision for this publication is that:

> **Communication and involvement should be recognised and valued as essential and integral to how we support people within services, across different settings, and by all individuals who support people with a learning disability.**

*Communicate with Me* is a learning resource designed to further the abilities of all communication partners to both communicate more effectively with people with a learning disability and to support people in a way which enables them to become more involved in their own lives (Figure 1). It is designed to support communication partners to meet the daily challenge to more effectively communicate with, and involve, the people they support. This resource recognises the requirement for communication to be tailored to individual needs and is both practical and theoretical.

Making positive and effective communication happen for people with learning disabilities who are supported in our services involves commitment throughout those services, from front-line practitioners and their managers to service managers. It also involves an awareness of the service's prevailing culture, and an honest assessment of how conducive to communication that culture is, a commitment to resources, an acknowledgement of the importance of communication as a human right, and a real desire to make a difference in people's lives.

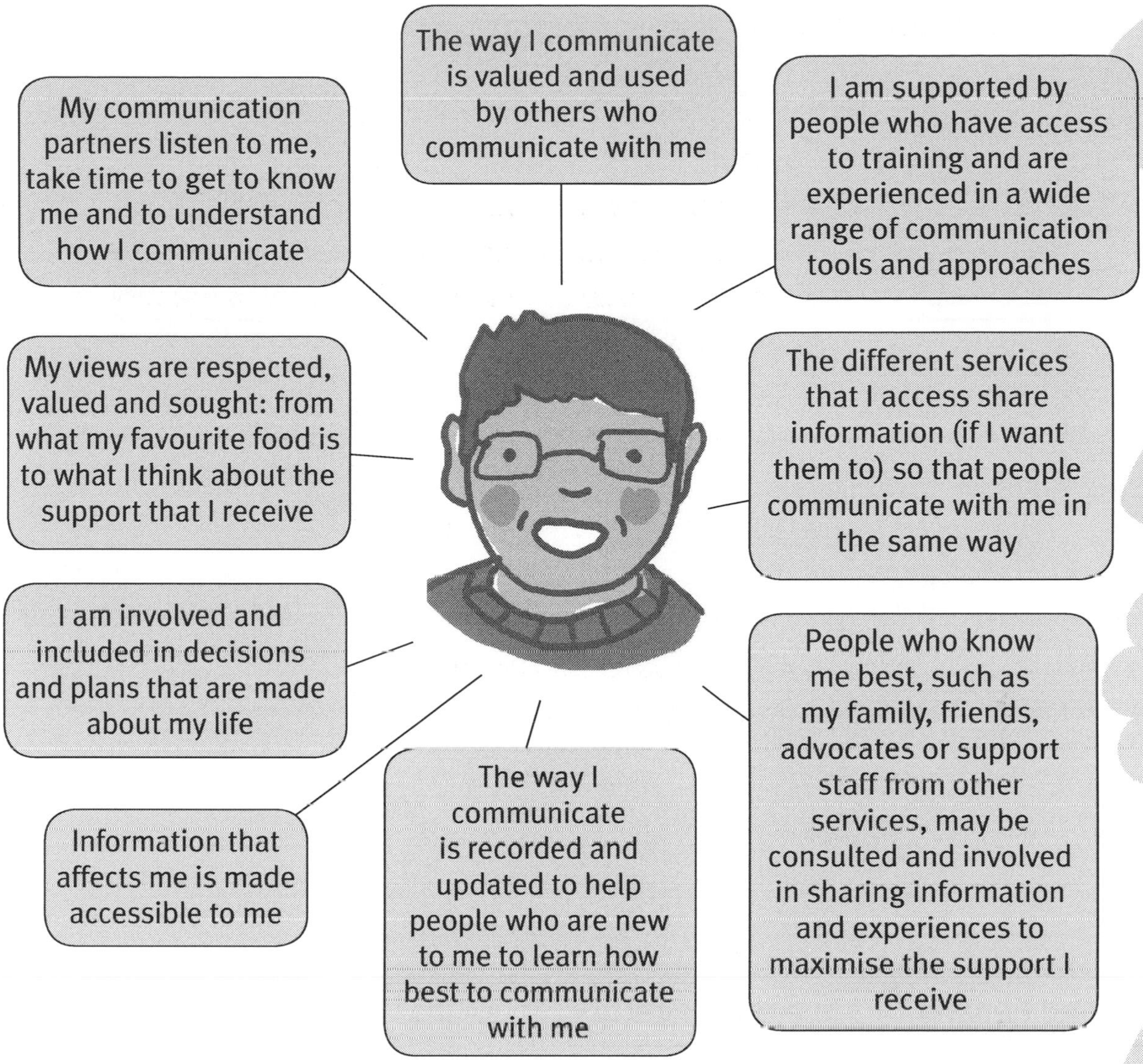

The way I communicate is valued and used by others who communicate with me

My communication partners listen to me, take time to get to know me and to understand how I communicate

I am supported by people who have access to training and are experienced in a wide range of communication tools and approaches

My views are respected, valued and sought: from what my favourite food is to what I think about the support that I receive

The different services that I access share information (if I want them to) so that people communicate with me in the same way

I am involved and included in decisions and plans that are made about my life

People who know me best, such as my family, friends, advocates or support staff from other services, may be consulted and involved in sharing information and experiences to maximise the support I receive

Information that affects me is made accessible to me

The way I communicate is recorded and updated to help people who are new to me to learn how best to communicate with me

**Figure 1** How a communication partner enriches the lives of people with learning disabilities

*Communicate with Me* is designed to support the whole service to consider and develop both how it communicates with, and involves, people with a learning disability in a way which enables change to become embedded in the culture and shared values of that service. This resource addresses the need for services to support communication both throughout the workforce and within the structures of that service. It also supports service managers to develop some aspects of the service to promote and support more effective communication throughout the service.

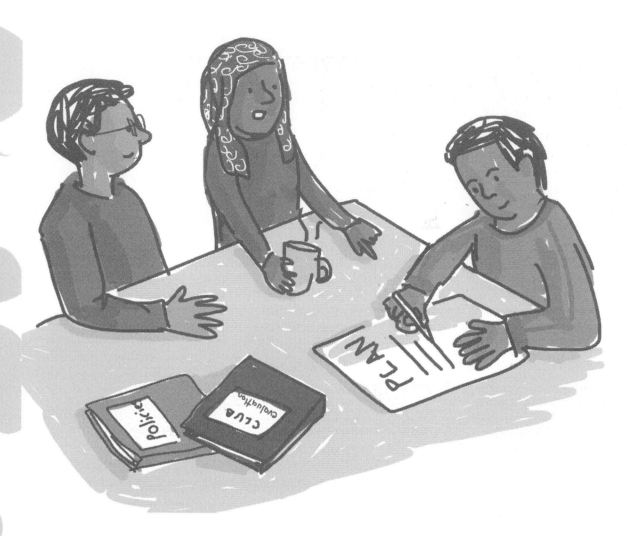

## The *Communicate with Me* series

In addition to this book, which provides guidance around communication methods and approaches, there is a *Communicate with Me* online resource which offers a Quality Assurance Framework to support services to implement good work practice in communication and involvement throughout the service structure. The online resource can also be used by individual practitioners to support application of the approaches. Please see details at the end of this book.

*Communicate with Me* has a website (www.communicatewithme.com) which provides further information and the opportunity for individuals and services to register their interest and/or their participation in the Quality Assurance Frameworks. Registration enables individuals or services to receive notification of training, future developments and additional services that may be of interest (please see the end of this book for more details).

Speechmark

# Foundation for communication and involvement

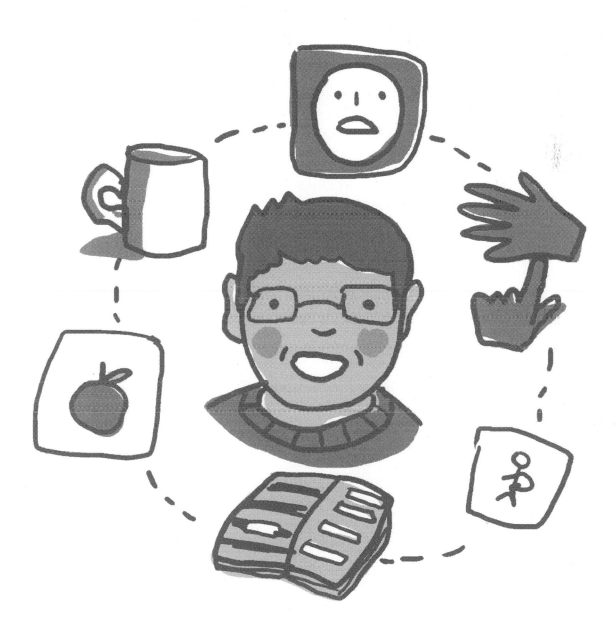

# Communication with and involvement of people with a learning disability

**'There are no people who cannot communicate ... just people whose language we do not understand.'**
(O'Brien & O'Brien, 1981, p62)

Currently, there is a range of support options for people with learning disabilities. Traditionally, the majority of people will receive support from services throughout their lives, to a greater or lesser extent. These services may include school or college, play and leisure services, residential or short break services, day services or supported employment. People may also be included in community circles of friends and other unpaid natural support. Increasingly, people with learning disabilities access personalised support which they may manage, with varying degrees of help from other people, as well as using a greater range of community settings.

The nature of support provided by each of these options may be different but all communication partners share the same challenge. Because the proportion of people with learning disabilities who experience difficulties in communicating is so high, the challenge is to effectively meet people's communication needs and involve them in their lives and their communities.

According to Nind & Hewett (2005), communication and the ability to socialise are the two human abilities which make the greatest contribution to a person's emotional well-being. They are the basic tools by which all else is achieved.

Therefore, how a person is supported to communicate and be involved in their lives can greatly impact on that person's quality of life. It follows, then, that the ability of the communication partner to support effective communication and involvement is central to an improved quality of life. The aspects of support for which communication and involvement are integral are shown in Figure 2 and in the following boxes below.

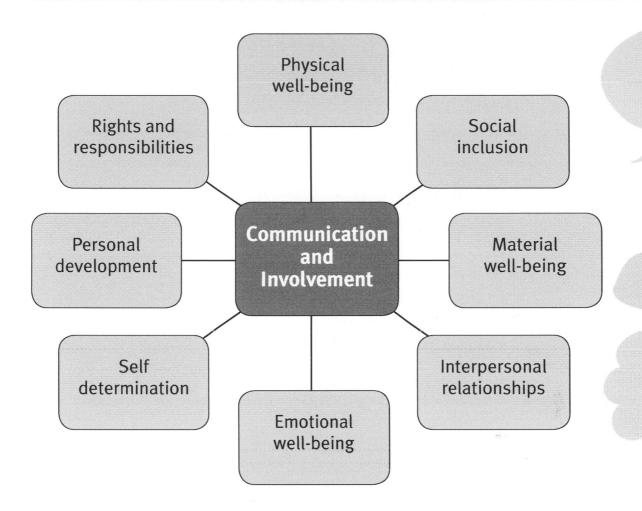

**Figure 2** Communication and involvement: integral to quality of life (*Source:* based on 'Domains and Indicators of the IASSID Quality of Life Framework'; Mansell & Brown, 2012)

## Physical well-being includes:

- Understanding how people communicate pain, discomfort and ill health; and supporting people to develop communication skills to express these.

- Supporting people to access and understand information about health care and well-being.

- Supporting people to make informed choices about health care, treatments and lifestyles.

- Supporting people to make choices and learn about nutrition and diet.

- Giving people the opportunity and choice to participate in exercise.

- Supporting people to understand what is about to happen; for example, going to see the doctor, what is involved in an examination or a procedure, how a person may feel after having dental work.

- Supporting people to understand when something is going to happen (this afternoon, tomorrow, next Wednesday, after Christmas, next year).

- Supporting people to follow instructions or guidance; for example, during breast screening, physiotherapy exercises, aftercare following surgery.

- Supporting people to share experiences; for example, giving an account to a doctor or making a complaint.

- Supporting people to understand experiences; for example, an accident or illness.

- Supporting people to make plans; for example, to follow a diet or an exercise programme, booking an appointment.

- Supporting people to understand change; for example, in body development, temporary or permanent loss of ability because of illness, accident or age.

## Social inclusion includes:

- Giving people the opportunity to take part in activities and spend time with others.

- Supporting people to experience different activities and to make choices about what to do and what to be involved in.

- Getting to know people and supporting them to get to know you.

- Sharing how people communicate so that others can communicate with them.

- Giving people access to their communication tools.

- Supporting people to understand their experiences and the experiences of others.

- Supporting people to share experiences with other people.

- Making plans; for example, inviting someone for a meal, joining a group, meeting with friends.

## Material well-being includes:

- Supporting people to make informed choices and show preferences about what to spend money on.

- Supporting people to develop skills in budgeting and saving money.

- Giving people the opportunity to use and plan how they spend and use their own money.

- Supporting people to understand the value of money and learn the skills needed to use money in their everyday lives.

- Giving people the opportunity to use their own money in everyday situations.

- Supporting people to choose their own possessions, furniture, etc.

- Supporting people to make requests about what they want.

- Supporting people to understand the material consequences of their actions; for example, how to save up for something, procedures such as banking, the consequences of spending.

- Supporting people to understand when something is going to happen; for example, a time line for saving up for something, that the new clothes will be bought on Saturday.

- Supporting people to understand change; for example, a reduced budget.

- Supporting people to access information; for example, statements, correspondence, information about purchases.

## Interpersonal relationships include:

- Giving people the opportunity to communicate with others.

- Supporting people to develop intimacy, trust and friendship.

- Sharing how people communicate so that others can communicate with them.

- Supporting people to explore and express who they are and what is important to them.

- Supporting people to share their experiences and to understand other people's experiences.

- Supporting people to understand change; for example, change in another person's behaviour.

## Emotional well-being includes:

- Supporting people to understand and express feelings, emotion and affection.

- Allowing people to express their feelings and supporting them by listening and responding.

- Supporting people to share and understand their own experiences and those of other people.

- Supporting people to recognise and respond to other people's feelings.

- Supporting people to understand change; for example, change in their own feelings and emotions or those of other people.

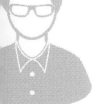

## Reflection

**For each of the areas of support listed above:**

1 Consider how people with learning disabilities might be excluded from opportunities.

2 Consider how increasing the effectiveness of communication and involvement may improve the quality of their lives.

The quality of communication and involvement in each of the areas of support listed above may significantly affect a person's quality of life. However, if the majority of areas are negatively affected, the overall quality of life of a person with a learning disability is greatly diminished. This often happens in a fashion where the person's quality of life and human rights are gradually reduced. A commitment to the communication and involvement of people with learning disabilities in all areas of their lives, even in a small way, will enhance the overall quality of support they receive.

One of the barriers that people with a learning disability encounter is the assumption that because a person does not communicate verbally, or has limited verbal communication, they are less able or even incapable of being involved in some of the support activities listed above (see Figure 2). This assumption can lead to a reduction in, or exclusion from, opportunities that people with a learning disability have to communicate and be meaningfully involved in aspects of their lives, which would lead to a reduction in the benefits of life-enriching opportunities available to other people.

Studies by Ware (2004a) demonstrated that people with a learning disability, especially those with profound and multiple learning disabilities, have fewer opportunities to communicate and interact with others. In another publication in the same year, she explained that responsive environments are ones in which people:

- *Get responses to their actions*

- *Have an opportunity to give responses*

- *Have an opportunity to take the lead in interactions.*

(Ware, 2004b)

Understanding how people communicate and having a range of methods and approaches available to support and promote effective communication is the key to overcoming this barrier. It is also the key to achieving positive support for people with a learning disability in all support areas in relation to Figure 2, the IASSID Quality of Life Framework (Mansell & Brown, 2012).

Therefore, it follows that communication partners need to be equipped with the knowledge and skills to support effective communication.

> **People [are] the most important communication resource ... People who value all means of communication, whether intentional or not; who take the time to really listen and respond; who are willing to nurture relationships and include those unable to intentionally communicate their views. People who believe in the human right of everyone to communicate.**

(Thurman, 2011, p14)

The skills and qualities of the communication partner can have the biggest impact on how effective communication is between two people (see Figure 3).

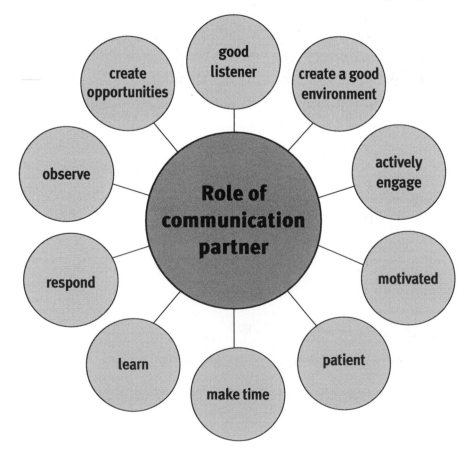

**Figure 3** Role of the communication partner

 Speechmark

# Communication: rights and responsibilities

Although there is no specific legislation regarding the right to communicate, the right to the freedom of expression is upheld by the Human Rights Act 1998, the UN Convention on the Rights of Persons with Disabilities (Article 9) 2006, the UN Convention on the Rights of the Child (Article 13) 1989, and the European Convention on Human Rights (Article 10) 2010.

Freedom of expression includes not only the content of expression but also the means of expression (Puddephatt, 2005). The means of expression that are typically discussed include writing, print, speech and the internet. But, equally, these means extend to other media through which people can express themselves, such as signing, using symbols and using communication aids (for example, choice boards), or indeed more subtle means, such as minimal physiological signs (for example, breathing or blink rate), or facial expressions.

The right to communicate encompasses the right to be communicated with in a way which is understood. This is represented by Acts such as the Disability Discrimination Act 1995 and 2005, and incorporated in the Equalities Act 2010, which responds to the needs of people to have information provided in accessible formats; and the Mental Capacity Act 2005, which prevents a person with a learning disability from automatically being excluded from being involved in decisions that affect their lives because they use alternative methods of communication.

Inseparable from the *rights* of people to communicate are the *responsibilities* of those who support them to enable that communication. In order to uphold a person's right to communicate, communication partners have a responsibility to explore and provide appropriate accessible formats to enable this.
Thurman (2011, pp13–14) states that to deliver this within settings and services involves an acknowledgement of:

> **The importance of communication as a human right and [the ability to] know how to support people to understand and express their thoughts, preferences and choices as far as they are able.**

As well as

> **A commitment to a co-ordinated inclusive communication approach from people at all levels – from families and direct care staff, commissioners of services, right through to policy and political leaders. It is a big task and requires both cultural change and a commitment to resources and real listening to people, however they communicate.**

## Reflection

1  Make a list of communication rights (eg 'the right to express personal preference and feelings', 'the right to be offered choices and alternatives').

2  Now, consider the people you support:

   • Do they experience these rights in the same way as you do?

   • What barriers do they experience in achieving these rights?

   • How can these barriers be overcome?

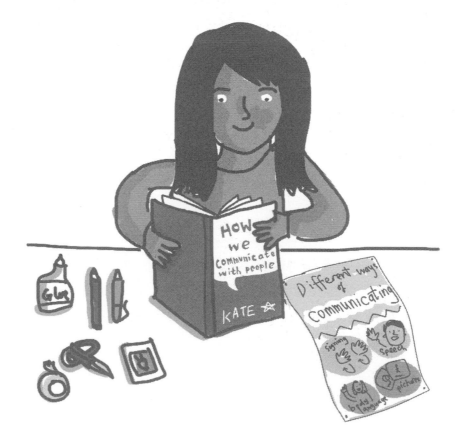

Through the above reflection, you might have explored a range of communication rights that all people with learning disabilities should have. You might also have considered how frequently these rights are not commonly upheld for people with learning disabilities. All communication partners share responsibility for reducing barriers to communication and enabling effective communication and involvement throughout their daily lives.

Those who support people with a learning disability, particularly paid practitioners, have a responsibility, both legally and morally, to uphold and facilitate the rights of the people they support to communicate (Figure 4). This can be achieved by gaining knowledge and work practice skills to support effective communication and by being able to apply this to all aspects of the support that they provide within that role.

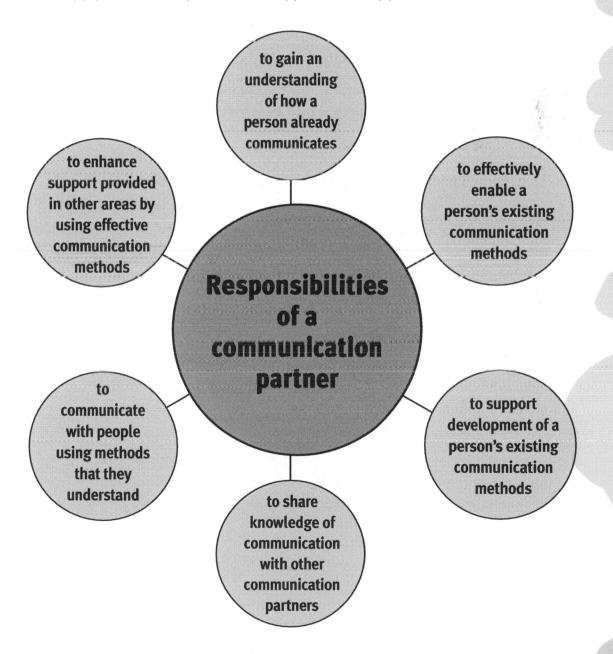

**Figure 4** Responsibilities of a communication partner

# Towards a culture of communication and involvement: medical and social models of disability

### Reflection

What do you consider to be good support?

Good support is ....

The commitment of communication partners to communicate with, and involve, people with learning disabilities requires the active promotion of a culture that is positive and empowering. It is also important for communication partners to consider how they view disability because this greatly influences the way in which they support people. The social and medical models of disability demonstrate how disability can be perceived and how society views disabled people. Attitudes and perceptions towards people with learning disabilities can greatly affect the communication opportunities and quality of support provided.

The social and medical models of disability were originally conceptualised by Mike Oliver (1990, 1996), Vic Finkelstein (1980, 1981) and Collin Barnes (1991).

## Medical model of disability

The medical model is a term that is used by some disabled people to describe how services and society most commonly consider disability. In this model, disability is considered in terms of the diagnosis of impairment and focuses on what the person has difficulty with.

The medical model views the difficulties that individuals experience as being caused by the impairment. In relation to communication, a person may be impaired in one of the following ways.

- Intellectual ability – ability to learn; concentrate; make associations; generalise; understand abstract ideas or concepts such as question words, concepts of time and emotional labels.

- Sensory skills – ability to distinguish between and recognise shapes, especially if they are abstract (for example, symbols, text or hand-writing); ability to distinguish between and recognise sounds.

- Physical ability – coordination; gross and fine motor skills. These may affect a person's ability to use sign language or form the required shapes for speech with their mouth and tongue.

In the medical model, support that is offered to people focuses on understanding and correcting these impairments.

## Reflection

1   Think about the people you support or have contact with. Consider the impairments which they have and how these affect communication.

2   How does knowing about the impairment help you to support people to communicate?

There may be a range of issues due to the nature of a person's impairment that make it harder to communicate. Broadly, these can include the above issues in the areas of intellectual, sensory or physical ability. A communication partner will need to recognise areas of difficulty that a person may have in communication and why they might find some aspects of communication difficult.

## Social model of disability

Some disabled people feel that the medical model view of disability is oppressive because the cause of disability is considered to be located in the individual and the impairment. Support within the medical model of disability focuses on identifying what is wrong with a person and correcting the impairment.

Some disabled people argue that, although it is important to have an understanding of impairments, the cause of a person's disability is located not in the individual but in society and social constructs. The 'problem' is no longer associated with the individual and the impairment. Instead it is seen in terms of the barriers that need to be overcome within society in order for that person to take part in everyday activities. If these barriers can be overcome, this means that a person may still have an impairment but is not disabled by it.

In the social model, support focuses not on a person's impairment but on identifying barriers and overcoming or reducing these. Some of the barriers to communication that might exist in services supporting people with a learning disability include the following.

- Lack of understanding; eg assumptions are made that people cannot communicate.

- Other people's reactions to disability affect how they communicate: eg pity, fear of how someone looks or sounds, disregard.

- Lack of confidence or experience (which may result in a person not engaging with someone who uses alternative methods of communication).

- Lack of guidance and support available to practitioners.

- Lack of training in communication approaches and tools.

- Lack of skills among practitioners and managers.

- Lack of creativity in approaches.

- Practitioners not taking time to get to know someone and how they communicate.

- Poor, or no, support plans which show how a person communicates and how they like people to communicate with them.

- Information not being shared between practitioners, teams and services.

- Inconsistency within the team.

- Lack of communication tools preventing a person from communicating in the way they are used to.

- Limited resources to support communication.

- Limited time due to pressures of work tasks, time spent communicating with people not being prioritised, or practitioners communicating more with each other than with the people they support.

- Lack of interest by practitioners.

- Assumptions made about what a person cannot participate in, is able or unable to do, about what they like or dislike, and their preferences or opinions.

- Political barriers: papers and legislation influencing the work practice of individuals and services; provision and allocation of services; control of funding for services.

### Reflection

1  Consider the people you support or have contact with. How might the barriers listed above affect communication?

2  How can understanding the barriers to communication help you to support people to communicate?

The concept of communication barriers helps shift our attention from a medical diagnosis that is based on what people see as wrong with the person to what we can do to better support communication. A communication partner has a responsibility to try to reduce the barriers that a person with a learning disability may experience in daily life and work with the person to support them to be understood and listened to. It is important for communication partners, settings and services as a whole to consider how they view disability and how this affects the way they support people to communicate and be involved.

## How the medical and social models affect work practice

It is important for individual practitioners, their managers and services as a whole to consider how they view disability and how this affects the way in which they support people. Table 1 overleaf outlines some of the key differences between the two models and how these affect both individual support relationships and service delivery.

### Reflection

1  Consider the difference between the medical and social models of disability.

2  Reflect on the way you, your team and/or your service currently support people in relation to Table 1.

**Table 1** Comparison of the medical and social models of disability (*Source:* adapted from Reiser & Mason, 1990)

| Medical model | Social model |
| --- | --- |
| Focuses on impairment and what is wrong with an individual | Focuses on ability and the barriers that are faced by that individual |
| Disability is located in the individual and their impairments | Disability is located within society |
| Support focuses on correcting problems | Support focuses on overcoming barriers |
| Support plans focus on identifying impairments and how to correct problems caused by the impairment | Support plans focus on what someone can do, how they already communicate, how practitioners can engage at that level and how other barriers to communication are addressed |
| People with a learning disability join in activities, routines and opportunities that are appropriate to their impairment | Activities, routines and opportunities reflect the ability and preferences of the individual or group |
| Disabled people are dependent on other people and services | Disabled people can be interdependent and independent |
| Disabled people may feel powerless and not in control | Disabled people become empowered |

© Martin Goodwin, Jennie Miller and Cath Edwards  Speechmark

## Towards effective communication and involvement

Money and Thurman's model (1994; Figure 5 below) is a helpful way of ensuring effective communication and involvement. The model considers the means, reasons and opportunities that people with learning disabilities have to communicate as equal and interdependent.

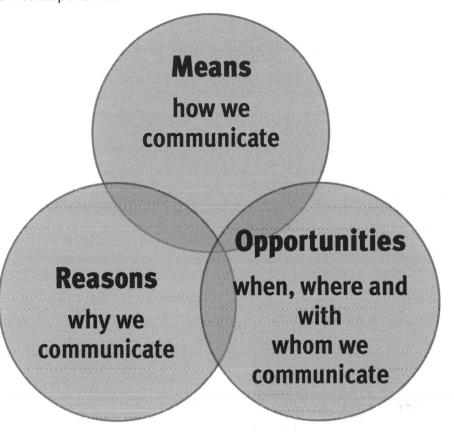

**Figure 5** Money and Thurman's model of communication (1994)

---

### Reflection

Think about a person you work with.

- What means does he or she have to communicate?
- Consider the reasons why he or she communicates.
- What opportunities does this person have to communicate?

Money and Thurman's model demonstrates that communication relies equally and interdependently on the three factors – means, reasons and opportunities. Take one aspect away and the person may find it difficult to communicate; to communicate effectively, all three aspects need to be equally considered and facilitated.

As Money & Thurman (1994) state:

- Without the means for communication, you cannot express yourself.

- Without reasons for communication, there is no point in or need to communicate.

- Without the opportunities, there cannot be any communication.

It is important to consider how people with a learning disability might find it difficult to express themselves and understand the world around them and to consider barriers that disable communication as well as the impairments that a person might have. An effective communication partner seeks to reduce or overcome barriers to communication and involvement so that the person's opportunities are not restricted. Effective communication is fostered through understanding how to support communication, enabling people's access and ensuring that opportunities for interaction are facilitated.

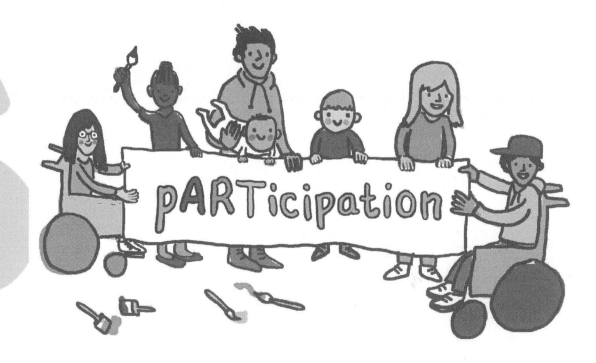

Speechmark

# Enabling effective communication

This section is in three parts. First, there is a discussion on the development of communication, including the challenges that people with learning disabilities may face, and a table showing the stages of communication development that people with learning disabilities may pass through, and the communication tools and approaches that are helpful at each stage. The second part covers a range of methods to help and support the development of communication with people with learning disabilities.

As Total Communication depends on the ideas in this section, it is discussed in the third part of this section. This involves identifying the needs of an individual and tailoring the communication partner's support specifically to that person's needs. As Total Communication depends on the ideas in this section, it is discussed at the end.

This section starts by considering the key factors that have an effect on communication and can make it difficult for people with a learning disability to communicate.

## Key factors affecting the development of communication

### Perception and attention

**Reflection**

Look at the pictures below. Can you see that the object is a plate? Think about how you know.

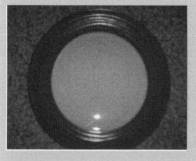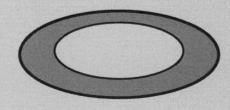

- Were you able to recognise the plate from the photograph?
- Were you able to recognise the plate from the symbol?
- Could you link the picture to a memory of the object without even trying?

You may be able to perceive the previous representations as plates, but please note: they are representations, not plates. Being presented with a real object is very different from being shown pictures. In trials, some participants thought that the photograph of a plate was a ceiling light, and that the symbol of a plate was a flying saucer; both are reasonable interpretations. Given time, though, most of the participants could interpret both images as a plate. They did this by comparing the images with their previous experiences of both real plates and pictures of plates. This can be a very difficult process for a person with learning disabilities because, while you may be able to call on the processes of perception, attention, concentration, memory and cognition to help you, a person with a learning disability might find these problematic, as the following case shows.

**Case Study**

Mary has learning disabilities. She is handling wooden blocks. She looks at the side of a wooden cylinder. From her perspective, it looks like a rectangle. Then, later, she looks at the end of the same cylinder. It looks like a circle. She does not realise that it is the same object as before, and she needs support with a lot of experiential play in order to form the concept 'cylinder'.

People with learning disabilities may not react or respond to environmental stimuli in a usual way or be able to control or integrate their experiences successfully. Perhaps the person finds it difficult to respond to sensory input or perhaps they over-react. Some people find filtering out unwanted stimuli difficult because all of the senses may compete against each other. This makes choosing what to focus on difficult or impossible. This is why it is important when communicating with someone who has a learning disability to make sure it is in a quiet environment with possible distractions, like the television, turned off.

**Case Study**

Ahmed has multiple disabilities. He is in a quiet room, being helped by an adult to practise his visual tracking skills. He shows that he can track consistently from side to side, following a torch beam. Other people are brought into the room; the staff with them are talking. Ahmed does not seem to be listening to the sounds, yet he stops being able to track visually.

Paul is being helped to drop a ball down a plastic tube. His communication partner is encouraging him to have his turn in the game by letting go of the ball: 'Come on Paul, let go!' Paul's hands clench into fists. After several more

> attempts to encourage Paul to release the ball, the worker stops talking and then co-actively assists Paul by gently using hand-under-hand. Paul is then able to concentrate on his hands and relax enough to let his helper assist him to let go of the ball. Paul finds processing information through more than one sensory channel difficult (in this case, auditory and physical – listening to the communication partner's instruction while trying to let go of the ball).

In the above examples Ahmed's and Paul's ability to concentrate was diminished and it is clear that they find it hard to attend to what is going on and to their communication partner at the same time. They are single-channel communicators and have not yet learned the skill of attending to two things at once.

Attention is a skill that needs to be developed over time, and it depends on the ability to receive and process sensory input. Ahmed and Paul were not able to simultaneously process and organise sensory inputs such as looking and listening or touching and listening at the same time.

For some people the ability to look or listen develops slowly and they may need much support and practice to attend to, scan and locate and prioritise visual or auditory stimuli in their environment. A person may also be hypersensitive (oversensitive and over-responsive to stimulus) or hyposensitive (undersensitive and under-responsive to stimulus) (see Jordan, 1999; Caldwell & Horwood, 2008). Hyper- and hyposensitivity can mean that a person needs careful support to ensure that they are able to communicate with you.

It is important when working with people with learning disabilities to bear in mind that attention can fluctuate for several reasons, including how the person feels and tiredness. The importance of an enabling environment cannot be overestimated (Ware, 2004b).

## Reflection

Go into two different environments which you attend with people you support. Close your eyes for a minute or two.

- What were you aware of?

- Did you manage to filter out any input, or prioritise what you wanted to attend to?

- Why might this be difficult for a person with a learning disability?

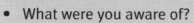

## Reflection

In the same environments as previously, do something you consider difficult, such as knitting or maths.

- Could you concentrate on the task?
- What stopped you, or what made it easy to concentrate?
- What might be the experience of a person with a learning disability?

In the above reflections, you might have realised that there are distractions in the environment that you hadn't noticed before. This is because you are used to filtering out (that is, ignoring) some of the stimuli that are not relevant to you. People with learning disabilities are far less able to do this, and are therefore much more prone to distraction or overload.

Please bear in mind, however, that although the above exercise may have emphasised auditory distractions, there are other environmental distractions to consider. Examples include an environment that is visually 'busy', or an immediate environment that overloads the sense of touch.

Getting to know the people you work with, and the unique needs, skills, abilities and difficulties they may have, is the first step in being an effective communication partner.

People with learning disabilities may experience the world in their own way. This is because they receive information in a different way or perhaps they find it difficult to organise and structure their perception of what is happening around them.

For example, there may be challenges in separating objects from their background because of perceptual difficulties.

## Case Study

Susie has a blue tray on her wheelchair. The adult places a purple ball on her tray. Susie does not respond. The adult places a white cloth under the ball. Susie lowers her gaze to it and stretches out her fingers to touch it.
The increased contrast of the white background helps Susie to notice the purple ball.

Another example is a person trying to understand a symbol on a notice board when they are distracted by several other symbols placed nearby. Similar problems can occur with other sensory inputs, such as when you are talking to a person with disabilities and the environment is not quiet.

Even the perception of everyday objects such as a table can be difficult for some people to process. For example, they may only recognise a table from a certain perspective.

## Reflection

Draw a table from at least three different angles.

- Which drawing is easier to understand and why?
- Why might a person with a learning disability have difficulty with this?

Many people may be able to perceive an object like a table in different ways and know that it is the same object. A simply drawn side-view of a table may confuse a person with a learning disability if it is not the drawing or representation they are used to.

People without learning disabilities can usually understand a wide range of representations of an object because of their more extensive experience, long practice in understanding symbolic representation and ability to recall and generalise. A person with a learning disability may not have some or most of these skills, or have them to a lesser degree.

It is important to bear in mind that even people with learning disabilities who appear to be able to communicate quite well will still need their communication partner to take into account their perceptual difficulties. For example, people who are beginning to read will need a font of consistent shape, size and spacing and the use of lower case letters whenever possible.

**Case Study**

Billy lives in a home for adults with learning disabilities. His communication partner is careful to create choice cards for him using lower case letters (as in the first example below) rather than with a capital letter (as in the second example). This is because it is easier to recognise the word shape.

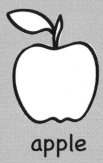

apple

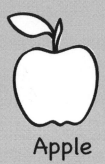

Apple

Maxine has been helped by her communication partner to make a book about herself using a computer program. There is space for more than one sentence on a page, but it helps Maxine to think about the meaning if she looks at only one idea at a time, so she needs to have just one sentence on each page (as in the example below).

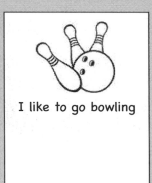

I like to go bowling

It is common for people with a learning disability to have difficulties with attention and perception. Perception difficulties can greatly affect the person's understanding of the world around them, as well as their understanding of symbolic representations of objects, in ways we may not always be able to understand. A communication partner may be unable to change the way a person is perceiving the environment around them, but they may support the person to a better understanding by giving cues appropriate to the person's level of communication development.

Attention difficulties can greatly impact on the person's ability to participate in activities and to communicate with other people. A communication partner can help by ensuring that the distractions in the environment are removed, or at least kept to a minimum, and ensuring that interactions take into account the person's ability to give or control their attention.

## Reflection

Think about a person you support.

1  What attention difficulties do you think they may have? How do you plan to help them?

2  What perception difficulties do you think they may have? How do you plan to help them?

## Memory and cognition

## Reflection

Choose an activity which you do at least once a week (eg using a washing machine) and see whether you can remember what you have to do. Then write down all the stages of the task. Think about the following questions.

• How easy or difficult was it to remember all of the steps?

• What prompts or clues do you use to help you remember?

• Why might a person with a learning disability find it difficult to remember the steps in an activity?

You might have reflected that some skills that you learn, perhaps after doing them once or twice, are quite automatic and you may be able to do them without really thinking about it. However, some people with a learning disability, such as Joe (see below), may find these skills more difficult to do. This is because they might find it hard to remember or access the information they need to complete the task.

## Case Study

Joe has been asked to wash up after a snack. He remembers to fill up the sink with water but the water is cold. He then puts the plates into the water but forgets to put in the washing-up liquid. To help Joe remember the steps, his communication partner takes photographs of the steps in the process and sticks them on the wall next to the sink.

In remembering how to complete a task, we may have to find a way of representing our knowledge and then link those representations together to form a sequence of steps. Often, tasks and activities such as washing-up or making toast and soup require us to simultaneously think about and carry out a number of actions. This is something that many of us are so used to doing that we don't even realise that we are using several thought processes.

The process of sequencing a number of steps or actions is a complex one for a person with a learning disability. In practice, the needed information may have to come from different parts of the brain because the person may not have clustered the necessary information together in a way that is easily accessed.

A person without a learning disability who carries out a new task or activity can draw on other experiences through a process of accessing memories and problem solving and be able to make sense of the task. People with a learning disability may struggle with taking in new ideas, words, thoughts, feelings, etc. This is because the mechanism in the brain that finds a place for a new idea among existing ideas (like fitting a new piece in a jigsaw puzzle) needs to practise many more times than in the brain of people without learning disabilities.

People with learning disabilities may find it easier to remember information that is presented visually or kinaesthetically (through touch). Visual information is more permanently available whereas auditory information, such as a verbal instruction, remains only in the hearer's memory, which can be a problem for people with memory difficulties (Kumin, 2012). Visual and tactile stimuli can aid the retention of information because they can be kept and used as cues. This is not to say that the communication partner should not give verbal instructions; just that it is important to be aware when the person needs extra cues.

People with learning disabilities may also find it hard to generalise information. For example, look at the pictures below.

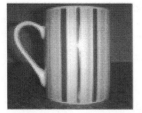  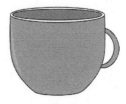

cup

Speechmark

People without learning disabilities may be able to understand instantly that the images represent a cup, but a person with a learning disability may not be able to. It may be, for example, that a person's concept of a cup is one with stripes, so when a cup is represented without the stripes, it may not be recognised because the detail has changed.

## Case Study

When Barry is asked to find a cup, he looks for a green one. If he can't find a green one, he thinks there aren't any cups because he hasn't yet learned that cups can be any colour. From then on, his communication partner gives him a drink in a different coloured cup each time. He also involves Barry in activities such as laying the table for a snack, repeatedly using the word 'cup'.

'Give everyone a cup please, Barry', 'Can you get the cups out Barry?', and so on, helping him if he is confused.

The communication partner also designs a card game that Barry can play with his friends, which involves matching pictures of a variety of cups.

The memory of people with learning disabilities is often shorter than other people's and they may have limited capacity in their working memory. This will mean that they can find it more difficult to locate and select memories. This then leads to the person being less able to recognise and understand the events around them and so feel less comfortable in taking part. For some people, each time they experience an object, a person or an environment it may seem like a new experience, especially if they have a poor working memory. For others, it may be that information processing is slow and they need more time for processing before they can give a response.

## Reflection

Think about a person you support.

1 What are some of their difficulties with memory and how do you help them?

2 What are some of their difficulties with information processing and how do you help them?

3 How does the person cope with generalising and how do you help them?

A person who is forgetful of people, places and activities or skills may be helped by being given cues appropriate to their level of development, such as the actual objects involved or photographs.

Problems with information processing may become apparent when a person seems to need a long time to think about things or 'take things in'. Their communication partner can help by giving them as much time as they need, and by making sure the person is not overwhelmed by information.

Difficulties with generalising become apparent when a person can work with one set of equipment, or in one environment, but cannot seem to transfer skills or knowledge. They can be helped by repeating the same activities with different objects, or by being offered, over time, different environments to practise in. Again, it helps a great deal to make sure that the person does not feel overwhelmed.

A highly significant stage in both memory and communication is the development of object permanence. This is when a person knows that an object or another person still exists even when they can no longer see it.

### Case Study

Mikey is playing with a rattle on his tray. His communication partner covers the rattle with a cloth. Mikey immediately loses interest and looks away. He doesn't know the rattle is still there. Next, the communication partner covers the rattle with a chiffon scarf which Mikey can see through. He is unsure. The communication partner encourages him to pull the scarf away by flapping the edge nearest to him. With many repetitions of this game, and similar games, Mikey begins to learn object permanence: that the rattle is still there even though he cannot see it.

The attainment of object permanence has significance for the development of communication because it allows the person to request or search for items that are not present. This greatly extends the range of potential communication, and it means that the person can take a step towards independence because they are not reliant on others to always anticipate their needs.

## Case Study

Sonia is thirsty. She is shown a carton of juice by a communication partner. Sonia recognises what it is and reaches for it. Another time when Sonia is thirsty and no one shows her a drink, she is unable to let anyone know what she wants. She does not know to reach towards the cupboard where the drinks are kept because she has not yet achieved object permanence and she only knows the juice exists if she can see it.

Mo has object permanence: he has learned to point to indicate his wants to a communication partner and he can also remember the location of significant items in the room. When he is thirsty, he vocalises to attract attention, then he points to the cupboard where the drinks are kept.

If people with learning disabilities do not achieve object permanence, communication will probably stay in a concrete form, eg using real objects (see 'Development from concrete to abstract communication'). The person is highly unlikely to be able to move on to abstract communication methods such as symbols or words.

With memory difficulties, the person may find it hard to follow instructions and complete tasks and activities. They may repeat the same questions or talk about the same thing over and over again. Difficulties with memory can also affect choice and decision making because the person may find it more difficult to choose from different options, especially when the options are not visible.

## Case Study

A communication partner asks Josh 'Do you want to paint?' Josh nods. He is given some paper and asked 'Do you want the green or blue paint?' Josh says 'Blue paint.' The communication partner says 'Do you want the blue or green paint?' Josh says 'Green paint.'

This example illustrates a tendency that many people have, which is to repeat the words or options they have heard. This is caused by difficulties with memory and the processing of information and meaning. Choices need to be presented in a way which helps the person to make a decision. For example as follows:

**Case Study**

The communication partner shows Josh some symbols on cards. Josh looks closely at each card in turn and, after several minutes, picks up the 'go outside' card, leaving 'paint', 'play with sand' and 'listen to music' on the table.

Here, a visual approach that uses symbols presented on cards helped Josh to understand the given choices and enabled him to link the picture to the concept. Staff would also have assessed that symbols were the correct tool for Josh's stage of development. As well as supporting choice making, symbols, pictures or objects used in this way can help with the development of communication and memory.

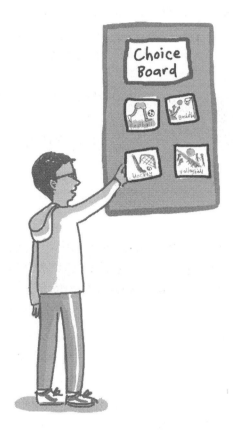

By ensuring that routines in the setting are predictable and repetitive, communication partners are helping to create an environment where people can best use their memories. In a setting where routines are more haphazard (eg meal times, break times), the person can feel less secure and more confused. An ordered environment allows the person to begin to recognise and anticipate what is going to happen and, therefore, have more opportunity to interact.

Communication partners can support people to communicate by ensuring that the early steps towards communication are repetitive and predictable. This will help the person to begin to feel a sense of control over their environment by being able to recognise and anticipate what is going to happen.

**Case Study**

To help John and the rest of the group know that drama is about to start, the communication partner bangs three times on a gong. Each person's name is then called in turn. When John's name is called, he bangs the gong to say that he is ready to join in. Then John is given a choice of masks to look at or wear. This routine is repeated in the same way at the start of every drama session.

Predictable routines help to foster a sense of security which, in turn, helps the person to feel more confident and more able to take part.

As an important part of the routines, the communication partners will use the same cues and prompts each time: for example, songs, sounds, symbols, objects of reference. It is essential, though, that the cues and prompts used are appropriate to each individual's developmental stage (see Table 2 on page 48) So, in a mixed group, several different cues may be needed or the use of an agreed shared cue to accommodate people's different stages of development. Cues and prompts presented through a range of communication approaches (as you will discover later) become a way of supporting people to be actively involved. Activities and interactions then support the development of communication and enable increased engagement and involvement in their lives.

A person's communication is strengthened by the opportunities and experiences that a communication partner provides. The process of learning through sensitively structured interactions, opportunities and experiences develops people's ability to communicate and understand. Observation plays an important part in helping people to understand. Through closely observing people, the communication partner can structure experiences that are intrinsically rewarding and motivating to the person, thus enhancing communication and interaction.

Communication and interaction should be sensitively supported to develop the beginnings of shared meanings and shared conversation in which two-way communication and interaction can gradually build and develop. It is the role of the communication partner, then, to make careful observations of the person to see what they are interested in and what this might mean to them, and to gently offer opportunities that are likely to help to extend their understanding.

Communication and understanding are inextricably linked and they develop in parallel, often through social interaction. All of the interactions that you have with the person are extremely important: they shape the person's understanding of themselves and the world around them; and the person learns that they can have a say and that what they say is important.

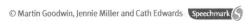

## Development of communication

The development of communication is complex. This section explores the areas of communication development that a person with a learning disability might find challenging.

### Development of receptive and expressive communication

Table 2, starting on page 48, shows the stages in the development of communication. While thinking about how the table relates to people with learning disabilities, it is essential to consider the concepts of receptive, and expressive communication.

> **Receptive language refers to meaning, understanding language and 'decoding' language.**
>
> **Expressive language refers to production, spoken output and coding – 'a process of formulating ideas into words and sentences, in accordance with the set of grammatical and semantic rules of language'.**

(Cantwell & Baker, 1987, p72)

In other words, receptive language is the language or form of communication that the person understands. Expressive language is the language or form of communication that the person uses. Receptive language is received from other people. Expressive language is how a person expresses themselves.

It is quite common for a person to be at different stages in their receptive and expressive language. Often, a person's receptive language is at a more advanced stage than their expressive language, although this is not always the case.

## Reflection

Think of a person you have worked with recently.

- What did the person appear to understand? (receptive communication)

- How did the person express his or her wants and needs? (expressive communication)

An understanding of a person's receptive and expressive language can help us to begin to understand ways in which we might more effectively support and/or develop communication. The concepts of receptive and expressive underpin all approaches. A person's receptive and expressive language development may be uneven because they may have strengths in one and weaknesses in another.

A basic assessment of receptive and expressive language, ideally with the support of an appropriately qualified person, is essential to the communication partner's understanding of how to communicate with the person now, and how to support their communication development. This will be carried out in conjunction with Table 2 which helps communication partners to understand the level of communication that they should be aiming for.

### Development of contingency and intentionality

An important stage in communication development is for the person to understand that they can have an effect on their environment. This is referred to as having contingency; that is, 'When I do this, something happens.' This helps a person's confidence with exploring objects, people and their environment and beginning to understand themselves in relation to their environment. Following this, people may learn to plan simple actions to produce desired results (a concept referred to as means–end). This should help to make learning and communication motivating for the person.

**Case Study**

Cosmo was tapping his fingers in a rhythm. The communication partner copied the rhythm in burst–pause modality in between the times when Cosmo stopped and also while he was tapping the rhythm. Cosmo appeared to enjoy this.

In the above example, Cosmo may well not yet understand that his communication partner was tapping in response to Cosmo's tapping. However, if the communication partner is consistent in responding to Cosmo's actions by joining in and copying, then Cosmo has the opportunity, in his own time, of beginning to understand that he can have an effect on another person.

The communication partner should look for every opportunity to respond to the person and help them learn contingency. The communication partner's behaviour can be described as 'acting as if', as in the following examples.

## Case Study

Amy's friend Asha is being helped to have a drink. Amy is intently watching every movement of the cup. Her communication partner says 'Want a drink, Amy?' and offers her a drink.

The fire alarm starts to ring. John is startled, cries out and looks frightened. His communication partner goes to him to reassure him, as if he had asked for help.

Some music starts to play. Constance smiles and starts to move her body from side to side. Her communication partner goes to her and takes her hand. He says 'Like the music? Want to dance?' and moves from side to side with her.

In each of the above examples, the person was responding to their environment without realising they were communicating anything. However, the communication partner 'acted as if' their behaviour was meant to be communicative. Eventually, the person may realise that their actions can have an effect on other people. When a person realises that their actions can have an effect on people, objects and the world around them, they may start to see a reason for communicating. But for some people with learning disabilities this is not an easy process.

Understanding the reason for communication is difficult for some people. Some will need explicit teaching that supports them to express themselves because they might not understand that their action is communicative. For example:

## Case Study

Jack went to the biscuit tin and got himself a biscuit. The communication partner asked 'Do you want a biscuit Jack?'

Here, Jack was getting himself a biscuit, an action which could be interpreted as communicative by Jack's communication partner even though Jack may not know that he is communicating 'I want a biscuit'. Jack's behaviour could have been seen as intentionally communicative if he had signalled his intent by pointing to the object while looking at his communication partner, or if he had made a sound while looking at the biscuit tin or said 'Biscuit' when his communication partner was nearby.

© Martin Goodwin, Jennie Miller and Cath Edwards  Speechmark

The act of asking for something – in this case, a biscuit – seems to be a simple one, but in fact it requires a set of skills. These include:

- requesting (Jack intentionally pointing or looking at an object he wants)

- joint attention (Jack being able to look at or point to the same object as the communication partner and being able to understand that they are looking at it too)

- alternating attention (Jack being able to switch his attention between an object, eg a biscuit, and the communication partner)

- understanding the social conventions of a question–answer format.

A communication partner can support the person to communicate and make functional requests by helping the person to:

- decide what they want, by helping them with a lot of exploration of objects, textures, tastes, etc

- learn that If they look at or reach towards something they want, such as when offered a choice of toys or snacks, then it will be given to them.

When the above step is well established, the communication partner may then be able to hesitate before giving the person their chosen object, so that the person has the opportunity to look at the communication partner.

When the person does this, the communication partner immediately gives them their chosen item. This stage requires a consistent and sensitive approach with much repetition. The person may then learn that if they look at their chosen object, then look at their communication partner, they will get what they want. Some of the people you support may find this difficult, but for others who can understand these important concepts, they are able to progress to more complex (increasingly abstract) forms of communication.

### Development from concrete to abstract communication

Familiarity with the stages of communication enables the communication partner to know how to support a person to develop skills appropriate to their ability level. For example, objects of reference can be used with people who are able to use concrete symbols to represent people, places or activities. Early on in this developmental stage, the objects selected must closely resemble the original. For example, an arm band or a swimming costume may be the object of reference to represent going swimming. It will not be the actual arm band or costume that the person uses.

'Concrete' communication means that communication is highly dependent on context and is presented in the here and now. To put it another way, communication at the concrete stage is largely referential.

In contrast to 'concrete' communication there is 'abstract' communication. Abstract communication increasingly uses more symbolic means of communication and is increasingly less dependent on context and situational prompts and cues. So, for example, a picture or symbol or word may be used to refer to going swimming rather than the actual object used. As Table 2 shows, within the category 'abstract symbols' there are several stages, from less to more abstract (see page 52).

The communication partner can help the person to progress from the concrete stage to being able to use more abstract objects. Using the above examples, a strip of the material from the arm band, or the air valve that is used to inflate it, could replace the arm band; the swimming costume could be replaced by, again, a strip of the material, or a badge that was sewn onto it. These new objects are more portable and an appropriate size to be used on resources such as key-rings and choice boards.

Pictures or symbols may also be introduced to support development towards more abstract representations. Initially, the picture would be shown to the person alongside the object. Then, after some time, the object would be gradually withdrawn. It is essential that these tools are effectively recorded, particularly when representations are abstract or individual to the person.

As communication develops, skills acquired in the earlier stages are often absorbed into how that person communicates. It follows, therefore, that people who are at any developmental stage of communication could also continue to use and benefit from the use of tools and methods of communication from the earlier developmental stages. For example, people who are able to communicate verbally may also be able to benefit from using tools such as signing, symbols or graphic facilitation to support communication.

The use of such approaches will depend on the need of the individual. Where one person might reach a stage of verbal communication and quite happily need no other support, another person may find verbal communication much more challenging, and will speak more confidently if they know they can use symbols, for example, if they need to.

The journey from concrete to abstract communication can be challenging for some people. They may develop increasingly abstract ways of communicating, for example, about an event that is in the future by using objects, symbols, photographs and/or words. More information about using objects, pictures, symbols, words and other means of communication is provided later in this book. For now, the focus is on the development of communication, mainly through speech and some other important concepts that help people to understand and use language.

### Development of speech

Non-verbal communication, which may or may not be pre-intentional, continues to be very important in supporting all people with a learning disability. An effective communication partner still looks for and recognises pre-intentional, unintentional and non-verbal communication even though the person they support may have more advanced communication skills. Picking up on unintentional and non-verbal communication can help staff to respond to a person in an appropriate and timely way. Examples of this are recognising the signals that show when a person's anxiety is increasing, which may lead to challenging behaviours if the person is not helped to de-escalate, or recognising that a person is feeling unwell or in pain. It also plays a large part in recognising and identifying serious issues such as abuse. It is therefore of utmost importance to be aware of, and to respect, all of the signals, both verbal and non-verbal, that a person may give.

As a person learns to use words, normally the first words used are nouns (naming words) or words that are relevant to the person's needs and wishes. People may gradually learn naming words (nouns), action words (verbs), describing words (adjectives) and grammar, often in that order. Before learning to use recognisable words, the person may use proto-words such as 'ron' for 'apron' and then gradually learn to link words, for example 'ball-out' for 'going out to play ball'.

### Case Study

When Hayley goes to the kitchen her communication partner asks her 'What do you put on?' and she answers 'Ron' for 'apron'. Her communication partner smiles and says 'Yes, apron.'

As words develop there are many conventions to learn which make the process of using language, both receptively and expressively, a challenge. Many of the issues that a person and their communication partner may encounter are covered later in the sections 'Development of grammar' and 'Communication breakdowns' below.

Communication partners can help in the following ways.

- Minimising distractions in the environment and making sure that the person can see your face clearly.

- Giving people time and space to communicate by not butting in, allowing people to make mistakes, but sensitively repairing their communication by asking questions, explaining and giving choices.

- Giving information in an easy to understand and simple way by avoiding long sentences such as 'Martin, it is time to get your coat on, the minibus will be here in 15 minutes' (unless you are sure that the person can understand this level of complexity) and maybe saying 'Martin, get your coat' or even more simply 'Coat'.

- Giving instructions in a logical order: 'Jamie, get your swimming things ... put your coat on ... get in the car'.

- Giving clear contextual cues and prompts as appropriate.

- Structuring sentences clearly and getting rid of irrelevant information or unnecessary words.

## Reflection

Read the following sentences. How would you make them easier to understand?

- Could you go and get the telephone book for me?

- Do you want a ham sandwich or a cheese sandwich?

Through this reflection you may have become aware of how easy it is to use too many words. The sentences are not particularly complicated, but they would be too complex for many people with a learning disability to process. Conversations and instructions can easily become cluttered with a range of unnecessary words. People begin by using and understanding single words, and their ability to understand an increasing number of words develops gradually.

1   At a one word stage, communication is largely referential, as much of the communication may be labels and basic words relating to the immediate environment.

2   As the person progresses to using two words together, they are more able to influence others and the environment by making simple requests, indicating people's possessions and describing actions.

3   At a three word stage, people use carrier phrases such as 'I want toast'. At this stage, people typically begin to ask 'What?', 'Why?' and 'Where?' questions, start to be able to maintain conversations, are able to express feelings (eg happy, sad) and internal states (eg tired, hungry), are able to assert independence, can talk about the past and the future and use plurals, with grammar starting to become more consistent, and can relate simple stories.

(*Source:* based on Kumin, 2012)

In addition, there is a development in the person's need to rely on situation and context. In emergent communication people are likely to have a situational understanding which means that they rely on the context (what is happening) more than what is being said. Charlotte Child describes this as a process of, first:

> **Understanding from situation rather than from words**
> * **Understanding equally from the situation and from what is said**
> * **Understanding what is being said.**

(Child, 2013)

A communication partner needs to be sensitive to the number of words that a person can understand in a sentence and the potential difficulty of some vocabulary. Using only a few highly relevant words at a time is known as 'minimal communication'. Some communication partners have difficulty with using a minimal communication approach because it appears to be too direct and perhaps not a polite or respectful way of communicating with a person.

On the other hand, remember that what sounds like a polite way of speaking to many people may well just sound hopelessly confusing to a person with learning difficulties. For example, it might sound polite to say 'I wonder, would you like the door closed?', but this could be very confusing for a person with learning difficulties. They may need to hear 'Close the door' and no more. It is important that the communication partner is conscious of the words they are using and adjusts their communication to the needs of their listener.

As language develops, an increasing amount of structure and number of rules are introduced to the person. It is important that the communication partner considers how they support the person with using and understanding grammar.

### Development of grammar

It is not unusual for people with learning disabilities to have difficulties with grammatical structure. Some examples are given below.

- Word order: 'Have you had a drink?' means something very different from 'You have had a drink'.

  Ways of helping: be aware that the person may use the wrong word order, and look for other ways of understanding their meaning, eg context. Gently repeat the words in the right order without making the person feel they are being corrected. Make sure that you support your spoken words with gestures and contextual clues to help understanding.

- Pronouns: there can be confusion between the words 'me' and 'you' (also 'mine' and 'yours') and, less serious in terms of meaning, confusion about when to use 'I' or 'me'.

  Ways of helping: avoid overtly correcting the person; this will make them feel they have said something 'wrong', but they are unlikely to learn from it. Instead, model the use of pronouns using puppets and in storytelling and drama, eg a story with a repeated refrain such as Jack saying 'I'm off to seek my fortune!'

- Negatives: it takes time and a lot of experience to learn that 'We are not playing football today' means something very different from 'We are playing football today'.

  Ways of helping: help the person to understand your meaning with your facial expressions, etc. For example, say 'We are not playing football today' with a sad expression and tone of voice and a shake of the head.

- Word endings that change meaning, eg walk, walked, walking and cat, cats.

  Ways of helping: rather than directly correcting the person's speech, repeat a more conventional version. For example, if the person says 'I walking to work this morning', the communication partner might say, 'Oh, you walked to work?'

- Longer sentences, that is, four words or more.

  Ways of helping: be on the look-out for signs that the person is struggling to understand. Try using simpler words and fewer words in a sentence.

All of the above problems can cause difficulties in expressing thoughts because they make it much more difficult to combine words into meaningful sequences that can be understood by other people. There is also the problem, of course, of understanding what other people may mean.

Another difficulty is that much spoken language is colloquial, with styles of expression and some words being peculiar to a particular region, town or even family. The forms of speech a person is used to at home may be quite different from the usual speech used by communication partners.

Where possible, communication partners should try to find out whether the language used in a person's home is different from the language used in the setting and make efforts to help the person to understand. This could be, for example, by incorporating alternative words. So if the midday meal is called 'lunch' in the setting and 'dins' at home, the communication partner could say 'Time for lunch. Dins!'

Understanding everyday concepts can be difficult for some people. Words such as 'soon', 'later', 'now', 'tomorrow' or 'at one o'clock' can be hard to understand and cause frustration because the words may be meaningless to the person.

## Case Study

Harry, who lives in a children's residential home, is looking forward to seeing his mum. He goes to his support worker and asks 'Mum?' (we think that he is asking a question because his voice has a rising intonation). Harry is told 'See mum tomorrow'. Harry does not appear to understand the word 'tomorrow' and shows excitement that his mum is coming. Later on, Harry returns to his support worker and asks 'Mum?' The support worker replies again 'See mum tomorrow' and Harry begins to slap himself.

The above case study highlights a difficult problem that is experienced in many settings, where a person does not have an advanced enough level of language to understand information that is important to them. This is a complex problem and there is probably not a simple answer, but an approach that includes good communication within the person's level of understanding, as well as sensitive emotional support may help. In Harry's case, the more secure and supported he feels in his residential home, the better he will be able to cope (see ' Understanding change' in Part 2). Harry's example shows us that language can be complex for some people to understand. Therefore, we will now consider the development of pragmatics.

### Development of pragmatics

> **Pragmatics – the skills which we use to interact effectively, share meaning and communicate with each other.**

(Martin, 2000, p10)

A lack of understanding of semantics (what words mean) and how the meaning relates to words (pragmatics) may mean that the person could get lost in the subtleties of language. For example, it may not be appropriate for a person with a learning disability in a work situation to call his boss 'mate' or to speak in the same way to his boss as his mates. People with learning disabilities may not know the social rules that are expected and may need support to understand social conventions and when to use different styles of communication.

We use language for a purpose and in a context. Here are some examples of the purposes of language, their potential for confusion and ways of helping.

- Forms of politeness: 'Please could you open the window?' means 'Open the window'.

  Ways of helping: it depends on the person's level of ability. A person who is just starting to speak and may use only single words, or at the most two words together, will be very restricted in what they are able to say if their communication partner insists that one of the words they use is 'Please' or 'Thank you'. These social graces are best left for later. Someone who is more advanced, perhaps stringing four words together, can begin to be helped to understand polite ways of expressing themselves.

- Jokes and humour: 'What do you get when you cross a kangaroo and a sheep? A woolly jumper!' (two meanings of the word 'jumper').

  Ways of helping: this example would be very hard to understand for many people with learning disabilities. Physical or 'slapstick' humour is often easier to understand. Try to avoid making jokes that people will not understand.

- Sarcasm: saying 'Well that's nice!' when you mean the opposite.

  Ways of helping: sarcasm is best avoided because it is hard to understand and potentially hurtful.

- Close-friends-talk: talk about personal concerns which would not be spoken about with other people.

  Ways of helping: chatting to friends about issues that perhaps cannot be talked about with others is one of life's pleasures and can be a valuable safety-valve for stress. Where possible, encourage friendships and provide time and space for conversations to take place.

- Formal language: less informal than the language used among friends, for example as used in an interview or at work when speaking to customers.

  Ways of helping: if a person you are supporting is going to meet a situation where formal language may be expected, help them to rehearse what they might say, through role play or drama.

(*Source:* adapted from Martin, 2000)

All of the above language purposes can be confusing for people with learning disabilities. It is important for the communication partner to get to know the person well, and to have a good grasp of their language ability to know how to help them.

Understanding what someone is saying it not just a decoding skill, it also involves the ability to see the other person's point of view (even if you don't agree with it). As a result of this, the person may adjust their communication appropriately. People with learning disabilities may find it difficult to make requests, alter the way they communicate, keep a conversation going, change the topic or cope with someone else changing the topic. People with additional impairments, such as autism, may find it difficult to read a social situation accurately and to empathise accordingly with the other people involved.

People with autism find it difficult to see another's point of view, but so do many people with learning disabilities. Failing to understand someone else's point of view, or even to grasp that they have one, is known as a lack of 'theory of mind'. Theory of mind may be absent because of the way a person's brain is organised, or because the person has a developmental delay and they have not yet achieved the prerequisites to develop theory of mind.

So what does a person need to have in place before theory of mind develops? There are processes of interaction which have been shown to be related to the development of social cognition, or theory of mind:

- affect, or emotion, and imitation
- the expression of desires and intentions
- joint attention to events and people
- pretence, play and imagination.

   (*Source:* adapted from Grove & Park, 2001)

## Overview of communication development

All of the processes discussed in this section can be encouraged in a person-centred environment. They can also be supported through communication partners who sensitively support interactions so that the person is empowered to understand their own and other people's emotions which greatly shape communication.

As you have seen, people with learning disabilities may or may not follow typical communication development. It is important that communication partners understand where people are in their development of communication and that the support offered is tailored to the developmental stage. This will help communication partners to make sure that they communicate effectively with people with learning disabilities by taking into account and meeting their support needs.

Table 2 outlines the developmental stages of communication in more detail with examples to illustrate each one.

**Table 2** Communication development and potential communication tools and approaches (Source: adapted from Rowland, 1996)

| Stage of communication/ development | Description and notes | Communication tool appropriate to stage | Case studies |
|---|---|---|---|
| Involuntary pre-intentional behaviours | People show only involuntary/reflexive responses, such as crying or blinking, to internal or external stimuli usually associated with well-being, eg pain, hunger. These must be responded to as if they are meaningful because without such a response from the communication partner, the person will be much less likely to progress to intentional communication. | Actual objects<br><br>The person is shown the actual object that will be used.<br><br>Intensive interaction<br><br>May be used to engage with people and to support development towards intentional communication. | Sasha has low vision and profound multiple learning difficulties. She is lying on a mat with a small silver torch suspended above her. She appears to fix her gaze on the torch. Her communication partner says 'Do you like that?' and sets it swinging a little. Sasha has not yet learned the skill of visual tracking but, as the torch passes across her field of vision, her eyes appear to widen. Her communication partner chuckles and says again 'Do you like that?' He stops the movement of the torch and waits. Sasha blinks. Her communication partner says 'Again' and sets the torch swinging. |
| Voluntary pre-intentional behaviours | Behaviours are voluntary but not intentionally communicative, as people do not yet realise that their behaviours can influence others. An example would be reaching for an object without realising that this action shows a desire for the object.<br><br>Communication partners should interpret and respond to these behaviours as communicative. Among other things, people may communicate refusal/rejection, a desire for more of an action/object, a desire for attention or a show of affection. | Actual objects (as above)<br><br>Intensive interaction (as above) | Winston has multiple disabilities including cerebral palsy. He is in his standing frame. He has a battery-operated fluffy dog on the tray. He is looking at the dog, then swings his arm around towards it, as if trying to touch it. His communication partner says 'More' and presses the switch that makes the dog move. Winston laughs.<br><br>Each time Winston moves his arm towards the dog, his communication partner responds in the same way. It is likely to take many repetitions over weeks and months for Winston to understand that his communication partner is responding to his arm movement. |

*continued overleaf*

Speechmark

| Stage of communication/ development | Description and notes | Communication tool appropriate to stage | Case studies |
|---|---|---|---|
| Unconventional intentional communication | People communicate intentionally but in unconventional ways, eg body movement. They realise that other people can be used to obtain something they want.<br><br>This is a highly significant stage. The person is beginning to understand that they can influence other people around them, and there is great potential for an increase in motivation. The communication partner's role is crucial in responding to the person's attempts at communication, and thus confirming that the person's efforts are worthwhile. Conversely, if the person tries to communicate and they get no response, they can soon learn that there is no point in trying and give up. | Actual objects (as above)<br><br>Intensive interaction (as above) | Dipiya is in her wheelchair. She is tapping her hand on the tray of the chair, while looking towards her communication partner. Her communication partner notices this, approaches her, smiles and says 'Sing?' He taps on the tray in time with Dipiya and sings her favourite song. |
| Conventional intentional communication (pre-symbolic) | People use pre-symbolic behaviours to communicate intentionally, eg gesture and vocalisation (but not words). The person acts on both communication partners and objects at the same time, eg gazing at someone and pointing to an object of interest to share their experience.<br><br>People at this stage typically communicate meanings such as: greeting others, requesting objects or more of something, | Actual objects (as above)<br><br>Intensive interaction (as above)<br><br>Objects of reference<br><br>An object is used to represent an event or an activity. It is not the actual object that will be | Dipiya has other gestures that she uses to try to communicate, such as patting her face when she wants a drink or waving her arms to show she likes swimming. Her communication partner tries to notice all of the communicative gestures and respond to them, as well as letting other staff know what her gestures mean and adding them to her communication passport.<br><br>Norman finds it hard to walk without help. There is a party for one of his friends in the home where he lives. Norman is seated at a table with some friends; there is a plate of sandwiches on the table, but Norman can see some crisps on the next table. First, he calls out to attract the attention of his communication partner, then he points to the crisps. His communication partner says 'Crisps, Norman?' Norman says 'Uh!' His communication partner brings the bowl of crisps and holds it for Norman to put a handful on his plate. |

Speechmark

| Stage of communication/development | Description and notes | Communication tool appropriate to stage | Case studies |
|---|---|---|---|
| | offering/sharing, directing the attention of others, confirming or negating information.<br><br>At this stage, some people will start to be ready to begin using objects of reference and may start to understand gestures that mimic the real action, eg running, brushing hair. | used in the activity. The same object of reference is used consistently. As the objects are real, but not the one that is used in the action, this is the beginning of the use of symbols, and it overlaps with 'Concrete symbols' below. | |
| Concrete symbols | Learners begin to use concrete symbols to represent objects or people. Such symbols may be objects, pictures, actions or gestures. There must be a clear relationship to the original object, ie the object selected must resemble the original in terms of appearance, feel, sound or action made. Usually, the person will remain at the stage of using objects of reference for some time before progressing to using photographs. The person may request objects not present and label other people or objects.<br><br>As the progression from objects of reference to photos to drawings to symbols is a gradual one, there will not necessarily be a clear distinction between this stage and the next. Some symbols can be relatively realistic, others do not bear much relation to the original item and simply need to be learned. | Objects of reference (as above)<br><br>Photographs<br>These should be clear, without unnecessary detail, uncluttered and in colour. They should look as realistic as possible and be of a size that the person can see easily.<br><br>Drawings or other pictures<br>These should be chosen to be realistic and easy to understand.<br><br>Symbols<br>These tend to be more stylised but can be chosen to be more or less abstract as appropriate. | Tyler loves playing football during his lunch break. Previously, his communication partner has been showing him the actual football that Tyler plays with whenever it is time for a football game. Now, Tyler is shown the real football and a small, soft toy football at football time.<br><br>This goes on for some weeks, and then Tyler's communication partner shows him just the small football. Tyler gets excited and points outside; he seems to have understood the small ball 'object of reference'.<br><br>The object of reference is kept hung on a hook on the wall with a loop of string. After several more weeks, Tyler goes to the object of reference, takes it off its hook and gives it to his communication partner. He is now able to use the object of reference to express his wants. |

continued overleaf

| Stage of communication/ development | Description and notes | Communication tool appropriate to stage | Case studies |
|---|---|---|---|
| | | Many settings use a commercially available program that represent her favourite things and activities to print symbols; this can have the advantage of consistency if the person uses two or more settings or services. | Macy has her own book of photos that represent her favourite things and activities that take place in her day centre. When she wants to listen to music, for example, she finds the photo of CDs, removes it from her book and shows it to her communication partner, who gets out the box of CDs and helps her to put one in the player. |
| | | Symbols can be used singly at first, and later combined, perhaps on a key-ring or by using the Picture Exchange Communication System, which overlaps with the stage below. | |
| Abstract symbols | Abstract symbols are used (eg emergent speech, manual signs, Braille or printed words, abstract graphic symbols). Learners may also have their own consistent patterns of sound which represent objects, people or events, eg 'Gorgog' for Granddad, 'bo-bos' for sleep. | Symbols (as above) Some graphic symbols are abstract and do not look much like the original item. | Lydia lives in sheltered accommodation and has been learning signing for the last year. While out on a shopping trip, Lydia slaps her right shoulder with her left hand. Her communication partner knows that this is Lydia's version of the sign for 'toilet', and takes her straight away to the supermarket toilet. |
| | | Emergent speech People often use speech at this stage; communication partners need to be aware of the person's needs in terms of both receptive and expressive language (see page 36) and tailor their communication accordingly. | Rookie has been using graphic symbols at school for some time and is ready to begin learning to read printed words. Her communication partner sits down with her at the computer, and shows her the program that combines symbols and printed words. |

Speechmark

| Stage of communication/ development | Description and notes | Communication tool appropriate to stage | Case studies |
|---|---|---|---|
| | | Manual signs (eg Makaton, Signalong) Signing has many benefits but one challenge is that because the signs are made with the hands, many of them disappear as soon as they are made, so the person has to understand them quickly or rely on their memory. | He asks her for some of her favourite things to do, and she tells him 'Swimming, dinner and dancing'. He types in each word separately while Rookie watches the symbol appear on the screen. They print out the words with their symbols and Rookie's communication partner helps her to stick them in a book. This is the start of Rookie's first 'reading book'. |
| Spoken and/or written language | Two or three abstract symbols (spoken or written words) are combined and learners begin to use grammatical rules (see page 44). The abstract symbols can be written words or spoken words. Generally, speech appears some time before the person is ready for written language. | Printed words (as above)<br><br>Handwritten words Handwriting is more difficult to read than print because handwriting varies between individuals. Cursive (joined-up) handwriting, especially if slanted, is more abstract and harder to read than printed handwriting where the letters are separated. However, as the person becomes ready, it is important that they have practice in reading handwriting as well as print. | Idries is sitting in a group for circle time. The leader asks what everyone did at the weekend. Various members of the group volunteer information and are listened to in turn. Idries is usually happy to chat one to one.<br><br>Today, his communication partner has noticed him looking at the leader and whispering a word or two, which has not been noticed. His communication partner speaks to him quietly, encouraging him to have his say. Eventually, Idries manages to speak up and catch the leader's attention, and then tells the group about going to a family party at the weekend. |

## Reflection

Think of two people you currently work with, each of whom is at a different stage of development.

1   How does each person communicate in relation to the stages shown in Table 2?

2   Now think about how you communicate with each person and whether this corresponds to their stage of communication development. Is there anything you could do differently?

You might have found it tricky to decide at which stage a person is functioning. It could be necessary to carry out several observations before you can place a person on Table 2, and you will probably want to talk to other staff involved with the person as well as their family. While Table 2 is not intended to replace the advice and assessment of a qualified person, such as a speech and language therapist, it should act as a reminder for you to offer communication tools relevant to the stage of communication development of the individual.

A careful consideration of the earlier section 'Development of receptive and expressive communication' is essential to a fuller understanding of a person's current communication development.

You may have found that the methods of communication being used with a person are not appropriate to the stage they seem to have reached. This will lead you to consider the tools and approaches that might be more appropriate.

For a person to move from one stage to the next may take years; for some it may not happen. Working beyond a person's level of understanding will not help them to develop, as it may confuse them and, ultimately, hold them back.

## Supporting people to develop communication skills

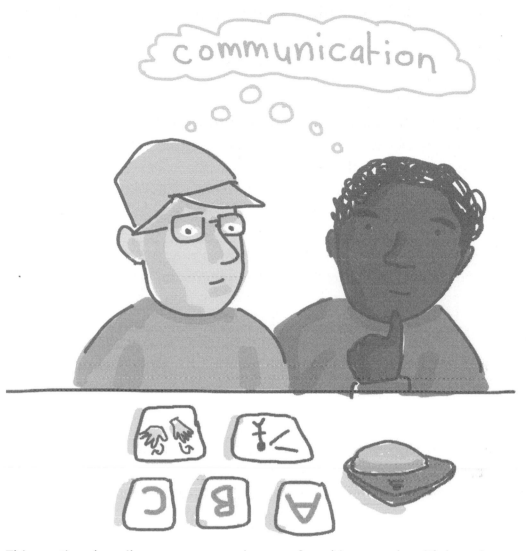

This section describes some general ways of working people with learning disabilities in the context of communication. While your role may not be to teach people how to develop their communication, it is useful to have an understanding of some ways of supporting people to learn. An important starting point is getting to know how a person communicates.

## Reflection

Consider one person you work with who uses little or no verbal communication.

1   How did it feel when you first met or supported this person?

2   How did you learn about how they communicate?

When meeting a person for the first time, you may have a range of assumptions about their communicative ability, perhaps from other people's opinions, or because the person reminds you of someone you used to work with, or based on the way they respond in one or two limited situations. Whatever your initial impression of a person might be, it is important to get to know them over time and in different situations.

When getting to know a person, the activities you are both involved in can make a huge difference, as involvement in activities often makes a difference to how the person communicates and what they communicate about. It is easy to base your initial opinions on your first interactions. A good communication partner spends lots of time getting to know the person through a range of activities.

Through developing a relationship with the person, and engaging in activities that are meaningful to the person, a practitioner can develop a more understanding relationship that provides a strong foundation for developing interaction and communication.

The 'getting to know you' process (Brost & Johnson, 1982) can be made more effective when key information is recorded about how the person communicates. For example:

- 'Emily understands and uses the following signs ...' (Here there would be a list of the signs that Emily understands, and a list of the signs she can use, along with other important information, such as whether she uses the standard signs or has her own versions, and when and where she uses her signs.)

- 'Alfie has a set of key-rings for making choices about activities; these use a mixture of symbols and photographs.' (Here there would be a list of the symbols and photographs on the key-rings, as well as an explanation of how Alfie uses his key-rings.)

- 'Ndhafa benefits from graphic facilitation during meetings and discussions.' (Here there would be an explanation of the type of graphic facilitation that Ndhafa uses, along with examples.)

Other details that are significant for that person should also be included:

- 'For John, communication is more effective in quieter environments.'

- 'When talking to Ollie, always face him and give good eye contact as he uses cues from body language and facial expressions to understand what is being said.'

- 'Neelam has a visual impairment and she likes you to be quite close to her.'

Speechmark

This information may already be available, or you may need to ask staff in other settings that the person attends or has attended, the person themselves if possible, and their family or carers. Having an understanding of how communication develops helps make sense of how people communicate and is useful in choosing the appropriate communication tools.

People learn communication best in a real context. If the person has learned to recognise a symbol, a picture or an object in more of a formal 'classroom' situation, ensure that you use the communication tool in a real context as soon as possible, so that the person can learn to use it functionally. This approach also helps to ensure that the learning has meaning and is useful to the person, rather than remaining theoretical.

Similarly, when deciding on the symbol, picture or object to add to the person's repertoire, consider what interests and motivates the person to communicate. Remember that communication is a social act as well as a functional one, so the priority should be to make it fun, interesting and meaningful.

When introducing new items to a person, consider using games, social activities, music and real items, as well as taking advantage of incidental interactions as they arise. This will help to involve the person and make learning meaningful and fun. As you say the word, link it clearly to the object, picture or word. Make sure that you use words consistently. These may be recorded in a communication dictionary or 'Words I Know' list, remembering that the list for receptive vocabulary will probably be different from the expressive vocabulary, and this must be made clear.

Avoid the temptation to rush ahead when introducing something new. Try not to bring in too many new symbols, objects, etc at one time. Always move at a pace the person is comfortable with, remembering that 'little and often' is usually better than longer sessions.

All interactions with the person should aim to empower them to take as much control of the activity as they can through supported involvement and simple choice-making opportunities. Enabling effective interactions means being a good communicator yourself. This means listening, speaking clearly using easy-to-understand sentences and words, at the right level for the person, and sharing conversation with them by turn-taking and pausing. Do not be too directive; allow the person to share control of what you are doing and allow plenty of time for the person to make their contribution to the conversation.

A communication partner can be an essential bridge to supporting the person to understand the world around them and successfully engage with their world as independently as possible.

They may do this in the following ways:

- join in with what the person is doing

- demonstrate an activity

- offer motivating starting points that encourage the person's interest

- comment on what the person is doing

- ask simple questions to help the person understand

- make sure that the person has the opportunity to communicate actively as much as they can

- show the person alternative ways of doing things that could be easier

- use 'sabotaging' so something happens that is not meant to and together you work out what 'went wrong' and decide how to put it right

- add surprise so that the person and communication partner work out what is happening.

(*Source:* based on Collis & Lacey, 1996)

## Using prompts

There are many contexts in which the communication partner may need to use prompts. A prompt is an action by the communication partner that makes it more likely that the person will succeed in an action.

Prompts should be 'faded' when possible, to reduce the likelihood of the person becoming dependent on the communication partner rather than acting on their own initiative. Fading means that the prompt is gradually reduced, and the person completes more and more of the action for themselves until, ideally, the prompt is not needed at all. Of course, the ability of people with learning disabilities to give their attention and concentrate can change day by day and hour by hour, so the communication partner should be ready to increase a prompt again if it is needed.

*Physical prompts*
This type of prompting uses respectful physical movement of the person. For example, when offering a person a choice of two toys, and after several minutes they reach for neither, it may be appropriate to physically help the person to explore each item. The communication partner could place their hand under the person's hand,

then place their own hand, with the person's hand on top, on a toy and gradually slide away their own hand, so the person's hand is in contact with the toy. If the person becomes uncomfortable at any time, the communication partner should stop. Prompting is meant to be helpful, with no suggestion of coercion. Once the person has examined both toys, they are better placed to indicate a choice.

A physical prompt can be faded by, when possible, gradually moving the person less. So, in the above example, when the person had become used to being helped in this way, the communication partner could place their hand, with the person's hand on top, only half-way onto the toy, leaving the person to complete the action. Then, over time, leave more and more of the action to be completed by the person, aiming eventually to perhaps just give a nudge towards the toy. The aim is for the person to understand eventually that they can choose to carry out the action by themselves with no prompt at all. Of course, if the action is not motivating to the person, physical prompting is unlikely to work.

*Gestural prompts*
The communication partner uses gestures to prompt a response in the person. Often, gestural prompts are used with people who are at a more advanced stage of communication development than those who need physical prompts. Clearly, the person has to be at a stage where they can understand the meaning of the gestures used. For example, if a person has two drinks to choose from, the communication partner may point to each one in turn, to encourage the person to look at each of them. The person may then be able to indicate a choice.

Gestural prompts are not quite as easy to fade as physical prompts. In the previous example, the communication partner could make their gestures smaller and smaller and, finally, just stand near the drinks without gesturing.

*Visual prompts*
These need to be something that a person can see, such as an object or a picture. For example, a person may have a series of visual prompts to complete the task of tidying away sports equipment. Their communication partner has taken a series of photographs of the steps involved, such as picking up footballs, taking them to the store cupboard, opening the storage box, placing the balls inside and closing the lid. The person looks at each photograph in turn to remind themselves of the next step.

Visual prompts are faded most commonly by reducing the size or the number of the prompts. So, in the above example, the person could be given smaller pictures or, when they are used to the routine of the task, the communication partner could give the person the first two pictures to help the person get started. The person then completes the task by using cues in the environment (eg when they are in the store cupboard they can see the storage box, which reminds them what to do). Of course, many people with learning disabilities, because of difficulties with attention and memory, will always need a certain amount of support with visual prompts.

*Verbal prompts*

A verbal prompt is something that the communication partner says. For example, if a person is sorting a pile of dirty washing and needs help, the communication partner could say 'Can you find all the white ones?', then 'Put the white ones in the machine and put the coloured ones back in the basket', and so on.

It is tricky to fade verbal prompts; you are either talking or you are not! However, the communication partner can try to reduce the amount of information given. So, in the above example, where at first the communication partner was giving instructions, they could begin to ask the person to remember more of the tasks.

The communication partner might say 'Now, how did we sort out the washing last time?', and when the white clothes are in the washing machine, they could say 'I wonder what we should do with these coloured ones?', and so on. However, if the person seems to be having difficulty with learning how to complete the actions without verbal prompts, it might be better to make some visual prompt cards, which they can use for themselves and have a degree of independence.

## Communication breakdowns

It is very common when supporting people with learning disabilities to experience breakdowns in communication. People with learning disabilities may find it difficult to comprehend what people around them are saying and they may show this by giving no response or an inappropriate or incorrect response. They may become confused, anxious or angry. This can happen when information is not clear or easy to understand, when they are asked questions, or requests are made of them in a way they find confusing, or generally during conversation.

It is most likely to happen in new contexts or where routines have changed or are different. A range of communication supports (covered in Parts 1–3) can help people with learning disabilities to be included, to communicate with others and to become more involved in their own lives. The causes of communication breakdowns can be varied. Some possible causes are listed below, as well as some suggestions for ways to help.

*Breakdowns in expressive communication*

- The person may be hard to understand. They may have problems with articulation, they may speak too softly or too quickly or have other difficulties with the physical process of expressing sounds.

© Martin Goodwin, Jennie Miller and Cath Edwards  Speechmark

Ways of helping: don't be afraid to ask the person to repeat what they have said. Always let the person know that you are interested in what they have to say, and never make them feel rushed. It may help to offer some supplementary forms of communication, such as encouraging them to point or using symbols. Never criticise the person's speech, even as a joke: a comment such as 'Come on, speak up!' can be hurtful. The person may find it hard to persist and tend to give up if they are not at first understood.

- The person may be shy, and find it difficult to communicate with someone they do not know well.

Ways of helping: any pressure to communicate is likely to make matters worse. Be gently encouraging and, if possible, simplify the demands of the situation.

- The person may forget what they wanted to express before they have completed the communication.

Ways of helping: it is very common for people with learning disabilities to have memory difficulties. Depending on the context, it may be appropriate to guess what the person wanted to communicate and make suggestions, or to wait while they try to retrieve their thoughts.

- The person may not be good at matching their tone of voice, gestures and facial expression to what they want to express.

Ways of helping: without being too obvious, model the desired behaviour by repeating some of what the person has said with an appropriate expression. Skills can also be taught quite naturally in drama, storytelling or social skills sessions.

### Breakdowns in receptive communication

- The person may have a sensory loss, eg hearing or vision, which makes it harder to understand another person's communication.

Ways of helping: the person should be accessing specialist support for their sensory loss; ask the specialist for advice and help.

- The staff member may be communicating at the wrong level, eg using symbols rather than objects, or using language that is too complex.

Ways of helping: make every effort to understand the person's developmental level. An assessment by a speech and language therapist is ideal but, if that is not available, try to find as much information on the person's level as you can.

Remember that a person's level of ability may vary from time to time and be prepared to take this into account.

- The communication offered may be at the right level but there are other distractions such as noise or a busy visual environment.

  Ways of helping: be aware of the surroundings from the point of view of the person with a learning disability. They may not appear to be distracted; rather, they may become more passive or, conversely, more active. Try going to a distraction-free environment and see whether that helps.

- Again, the communication may be at the right level but the person may be feeling upset or unwell.

  Ways of helping: the importance of getting to know the people you are working with cannot be overestimated. The better you know someone, the better you will be able to tell whether they are out of sorts.

- The person may have forgotten some previous knowledge, eg they used to know the symbol for 'cake' but, because they haven't used it in a while, they now cannot choose between a biscuit symbol and a cake symbol.

  Ways of helping: if this seems to be an issue for the person, agree a list of the most useful symbols (or objects of reference, or words) and try to use them frequently. Be prepared to offer help by matching the symbol to a real object, or by using more easily understood tools, such as photographs.

- The person may not be good at reading tone of voice, gestures and facial expressions and so misunderstands spoken words.

  Ways of helping: keep words and sentences simple, and say what you mean; that is, avoid sarcasm or jokey ways of communicating. Appropriate tone of voice, gestures and facial expressions can be explored and discussed in drama, storytelling or social skills sessions.

- The person may have a problem with short-term auditory memory; that is, the memory used to process spoken language. This makes it harder for them to listen to and recall the spoken word.

  Ways of helping: it may be enough to speak clearly and use very short sentences and simple words, or it may be necessary to further support your verbal communication with symbols or pictures.

Speechmark

Of course, there is a strong link between expressive and receptive communication, and most of the causes of communication breakdown can affect both. The lists above are not exhaustive, and you can probably think of other possible causes and, indeed, ways of helping.

## Reflection

Think of two or three people you work with.

1   How do you help each person to repair communication breakdowns?

2   How do you try to avoid communication breakdowns happening?

You might have reflected that communication breakdowns happen quite often and that this is an inevitable part of communication. After all, how many people (without a learning disability) always understand others, or always make themselves clear enough for other people to understand?

Some people with learning disabilities may be very good at letting you know that you have misunderstood them; others may need significant support and a communication partner they can trust, so they become confident in correcting miscommunication. Other people may rightly rely on your communication being correct and appropriate and it is your responsibility to make sure that you communicate as much as possible in the way a person can understand.

When you start working with a person, it is well worth seeing whether they have a communication profile, a communication passport or a report written by a speech and language therapist. If not, you could ask the person and those closely involved in the person's life if you could access a speech and language assessment and/or support for the person  Involving a speech and language therapist, if possible, will help you to tailor all of the communication tools and approaches outlined in the rest of this book.

This section explored several concepts and approaches that it is important to understand when enabling communication with people who have learning disabilities. In considering some important stages of how communication develops and how we can support communication, we now return to the concept of Total Communication.

## Total Communication

Total Communication is defined as:

> **a communication philosophy – not a communication method and not at all a teaching method ... Total Communication is an approach to create a successful and equal communication between human beings with different language perception and/or production.**

(Hansen, 1980, p5)

Total Communication covers a range of potential approaches and ways of communicating with people with a learning disability. Total Communication is about communicating in a variety of ways to enable more effective communication, while bearing in mind the person's level of communication development.

Therefore, Total Communication requires the communication partner to be aware of:

- the person's current ability within both expressive and receptive communication

- the effects of any barriers to communication, either permanent or temporary, that the person may be experiencing

- the possible causes of communication breakdowns, both within the person and in the environment, and ways of minimising them

- the person's personality and how this may affect their communication style

- any signals that the person may give at any time which indicate their mood and how relaxed and confident, or otherwise, they may be feeling

- any other information which may have an effect on communication, whether from the person themselves or from someone else.

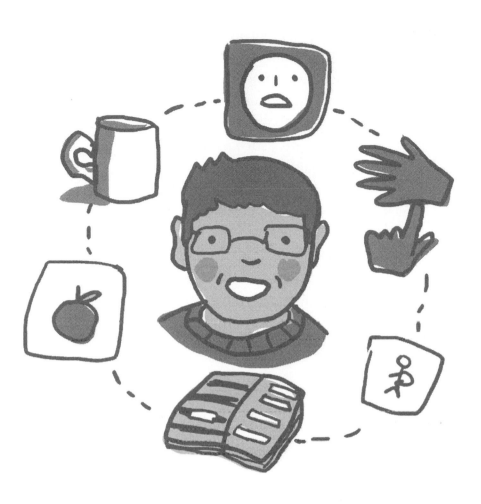

### Reflection

1  List as many different ways to communicate and as many tools to support communication as you can think of.

2  Consider some of the people you support. Identify the ways in which they communicate and which communication methods and tools you can use to communicate with them.

In the previous reflection you might have easily listed a range of different tools and approaches that you use to communicate with and involve people with a learning disability. Through talking to others, and finding out about the communication tools and approaches covered in Parts 1–3, you may become more aware of the range of communication tools and approaches that can be used. Perhaps you included in your list some of the less obvious 'tools', such as 'facial expression', 'tone of voice' or 'approachability, a welcoming manner'.

Reflection on your use of the range of different ways in which you can communicate and involve people with a learning disability is essential to effective communication and involvement. For example, you may find that you use a range of communication approaches but need to improve your understanding of them. Alternatively, you may find that there is an approach, which you are not yet using, that might help a person you support. Sharing information about how you communicate and your thoughts about communication will support both your own development and that of other communication partners.

### Case Study

Shugra has multiple needs. At dinner time, her communication partner shows her the dinner object of reference and says 'Dinner'. Shugra does not respond. Her communication partner shows her the object of reference again and says 'Dinner' in a bright tone and with a smile. Shugra looks up and smiles.

In the above example, the communication partner's facial expression and tone of voice may not have helped Shugra to understand the meaning of the object. However, in sounding interested and involved, the communication partner was helping her to engage with the object, and possibly communicating that 'dinner' is something to be pleased about.

### Case Study

In supported living, Barry is having a conversation with his communication partner, who is standing at the kitchen sink washing the dishes. After a while, Barry says less and less and, finally, he goes to his communication partner, takes her arm and turns her away from the sink, so that they can see each other's face while they talk.

Barry is capable of expressing himself through speech, and of understanding speech, but he needs the extra support of being able to see the person's facial expression and of knowing that the other person can see him. He starts to feel unsure and unsettled if he cannot do this.

**Case Study**

In a day care setting, part of the welcome board in the home room is an area where, on arrival, people can find their own Velcro-backed photo and move it to the 'I'm here!' area of the board. Hardeep's communication partner notices that, while Hardeep can recognise and choose his own photo if he is seated at a table on his own, he seems to get flustered when he is standing by the door and other people are coming in around him, and can't decide which photo is his. In consultation with the other staff members, Hardeep's communication partner makes a photo board that is separate from the welcome board and a few feet away, where there is less bustle. Hardeep is then able to find his photo and return to fix it to the welcome board.

In the above example, the stress that Hardeep felt in a busy area was preventing him from being able to use a communication aid which he would otherwise use easily. It was his communication partner's sensitive response to his observation of Hardeep that enabled Hardeep to complete the task.

Total Communication reflects the ways in which we all communicate. As Barbour (1976) demonstrated, the information we receive during a conversation with someone is made up of a variety of methods of communication. We draw meaning from people's facial expressions, their gestures, tone of voice, volume of speech and physical posture as well as the actual words that are spoken.

These layers of communication mean that if there are times when some of this information is missing, people without learning disabilities can fill in the gaps. For example, if there is a lot of background noise, people without learning disabilities, perhaps not realising they are doing it, watch people's lips more when they are talking and rely more on gestures and facial expression to fill in any gaps.

Sometimes, especially in the case of people without learning disabilities, the more layers of communication we can offer someone, the more effective our communication becomes. However, some people with a learning disability may only use one form of communication at a time (single-channel processing) or may only communicate in one way. Most importantly, people with a learning disability can often only access communication in the way they need to with the support of communication partners who can adapt and respond to the person's individual ways of communicating.

Total Communication is about recognising that a person with a learning disability may communicate in a range of different ways. All of these methods of communication should be respected and acknowledged, and communication partners should respond to the variety of communication needs through a range of relevant tools and approaches. The rest of this book is designed to help you find those tools and approaches.

---

## Reflection

1 What are the key things that you feel are important to make sure that communication is effective?

2 What would be the impact on a person with a learning disability if these key things are not in place?

---

Through this reflection you might have explored a range of values that support your ability to communicate and involve people with a learning disability. As discussed earlier, your values actively shape your interactions and influence the communication opportunities available to people with learning disabilities.

In practice, you may find that while you have values about communication with, and the involvement of, people with learning disabilities, you may find it hard to put them into practice. Once again, reflection on your own and others' values and ongoing discussions about how to put them into practice will help you to ensure effective communication and involvement.

In thinking about your values it is also important to commit to working to the values of the person whom you are supporting and to ensure that you are person-centred (see the section on person-centred planning in Part 2).

Total Communication uses communication methods and tools to further increase opportunities to positively engage with and involve people. These include: signing, using pictures and symbols, graphic facilitation, Intensive Interaction, key-rings, visual timetables and objects of reference. No one approach is better than any other because it is all about meeting the person's communication needs and one approach certainly would not suit all people. The tools and approaches have to be developed or learned by communication partners and may require additional resources.

Communication specialists such as speech and language therapists can help assess and advise communication approaches and strategies that may support the development of communication. As communication partners develop their skills and knowledge, the people they support will have greater opportunities to explore a wider range of options to express themselves and understand the world around them.

## Reflection

Ask someone to observe you when you are doing an activity or interacting with a person with a learning disability on two separate occasions. Ask them to give you feedback on how you:

- communicated and interacted with the person

- helped the person to have some control within the interaction

- helped the interaction to be two-way

- developed the quality of the interaction.

A commitment to reflection on communicating and involving people with a learning disability is one of the most important things that a communication partner can do. Ongoing reflection on the support you are offering will help you to understand and continually improve the way you shape your communication.

Remember that, in addition to a genuine commitment and desire to communicate with and involve the person, good communication and involvement take time and practice. More information about keeping up to date and improving your practice is included and integrated in this book, in particular in Part 3 on structuring for communication.

## Reflection

Take a look at the case studies below and answer the questions on them.

1   You support Rochelle at her home. She is able to understand some objects of reference but does not yet use them to communicate her wishes. She does not always appear to listen, or have a long attention span, and says 'Yes' in response to much of what you ask. She does seem to be able to see and hear quite well.

- How could you support Rochelle more effectively to make choices?

- For example, what colour would she like her room painted? Where would she like to go on a day out? What would she like to eat?

2   You are working in a supported tenancy which is staffed by a team who work shifts. The men you support are at an 'abstract symbolic' stage of development; they all understand some symbols and most of them understand simple speech. They all like to know who is working and when, sometimes days in advance.

- How could your team make this information accessible to them?

3   You are supporting a teenager to engage in some new activities. He is at a 'conventional intentional' stage of expressive development but does not yet understand symbols or speech.

- How could you support him to express whether he enjoyed himself or not and if he would like to do the activity again?

4   Every person who attends the school where you work receives an annual review. The service supports people with a range of communication support needs, from those who have some verbal communication to people who do not yet have intentional communication.

- Imagine three individuals with different support needs. How could you support them to be involved in both contributing to the review and being involved in the review on the day?

The case studies above represent a selection of issues that communication partners working in a variety of contexts may encounter. A communication partner's task is to get to know each person and then, with the person's involvement, to explore a range of approaches that will support the person to communicate and be involved as much as they can and want.

The rest of this book explores a range of different approaches that can be used in various contexts to support you in your commitment to improving your communication with and involvement of people with a learning disability.  The following sections are a learning resource that can be tailored to the individual needs of the person who is being supported, the learning needs of communication partners and/or the learning needs of a setting or service. The resource provides an introduction to a wide range of communication methods and tools to enhance work practice in areas of communication that are encountered on a daily basis as well as some that are more specific to different settings and services.

This resource can be used either independently or as part of a more structured training approach in conjunction with the interactive Quality Assurance Framework which is available in the online resource.

# *Communicate with Me* approaches and tools for work practice

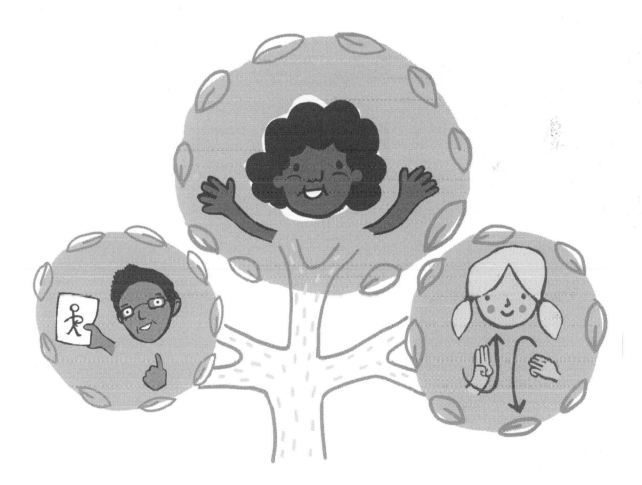

# Part 1
# Welcome me

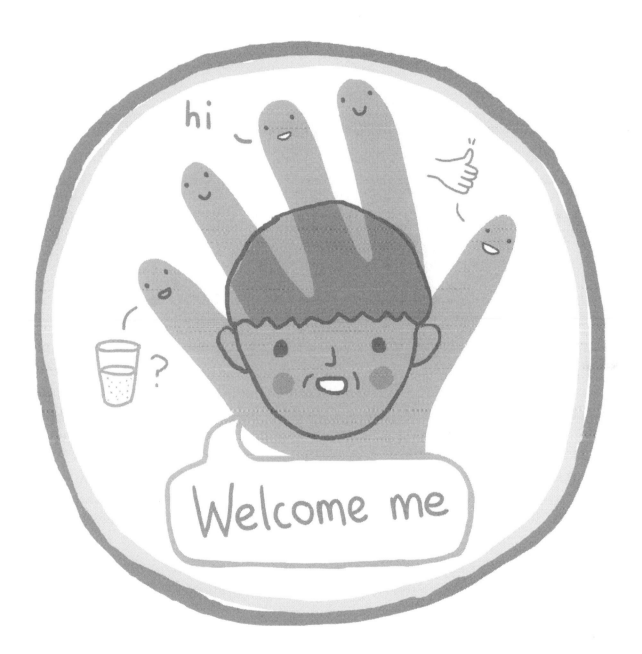

This part provides a set of tools to enable communication partners and services to promote a positive environment to establish and actively promote communication and involvement with people who have a learning disability.

# Welcome board

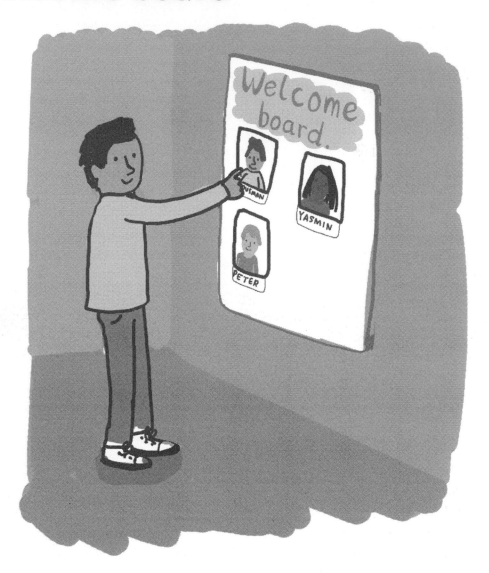

A welcome board is one of the first things that people see when they enter a setting. What is on the board should be tailored specifically to the needs of the people who access it and the activities or support that are provided. The message that is conveyed is 'welcome' and this can be the first opportunity to make someone feel valued when they enter an environment whether it is a day service, classroom or youth club. The board should be accessible to the communication needs of the people who use the setting. This can be achieved using an extensive range of communication methods, including words, symbols, photos and objects to enable people to understand it.

Welcome boards support people with a learning disability to make the conceptual link with the function of the environment. For example, what activities take place in a day service or the staff team in a short break house, or an introduction to an individual worker.

 **Speechmark**

Welcome boards can be a really creative project to introduce a service or setting to individuals or to welcome a specific individual to the start of a session. Think creatively about the format of the welcome board – it could be a traditional notice board in an entrance to a setting; or it could be a display table with tactile objects, photographs of the staff team or pictures of activities that take place in a setting. A welcome board can also be produced in other formats such as an accessible register, book or a profile.

## Reflection

1   When would a welcome board be useful? Consider two individuals who you support and discuss how a welcome board would be beneficial to them.

2   What information could be displayed on a welcome board?

3   How would you make sure that the welcome board is accessible to the people you support?

## Examples of good practice

A day service has a welcome board in the entrance hall. It has 'Welcome' in clear writing across the top. Underneath there are photographs of people who access the day service, engaging in activities such as the Christmas party, bowling, gardening, art and the monthly disco. A collage for each activity is made up of photographs, drawings, objects (such as dried flowers, theatre tickets or party streamers) and some writing. The collages are mounted on coloured sugar paper and evenly spaced out across the board. The board has a plain background so that it is not too busy. The welcome board is updated regularly by the people who access the day service.

Frank supports people to access leisure activities in the community. He uses a welcome file when he meets people for the first time. The first part of the file introduces himself and includes some photographs, pictures and a collage to show who he is, what is important to him and what he enjoys doing. The second part of the file includes some photographs of the sort of things that Frank supports other people to do. This part has been written with some of the people he supports as part of an activity or over a cup of coffee. Frank asked people what they liked about their support time, what they enjoyed doing and, with their permission, included some photographs of a few of these activities. Using the file helps Frank to build a relationship with new people who he supports.

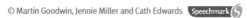

A play group for children with learning disabilities uses the welcome board for children to sign themselves in to the provision – children are supported to use a pen or stamp next to their photograph. The children can see who is there and which staff will be supporting them.

A museum has a welcome board that is situated in the reception of the building. The welcome board is for everyone who visits the museum but it has been made accessible to people with learning disabilities and other impairments. It displays tactile objects which communicate the theme of exhibition.

# Visual timetable

Visual timetables (which may also be called visual schedules, picture schedules or activity schedules) are used to show the order of events, routines or activities. Not knowing what is going to happen or who is going to support a person can be a source of anxiety for people with a learning disability. Having a timetable with information on it that people can access themselves can help people to feel more in control and can increase their independence.

Visual timetables can be presented in a chain (on a board from left to right or top to bottom) or a grid with several sections as appropriate. The timetable can be a fixed one, for example a school timetable, or it can be made to be changed daily using Velcro™ tabs or Blu Tack™. The timetable can concentrate on a specific time of the day (for example morning) or an activity such as going out into the community and returning to home.

As well as presenting routines to people, visual timetables can also be used to support people to plan activities for that day or for the week themselves. This can be achieved by supporting a person to choose symbols or pictures of activities and then fixing them to the timetable in the appropriate space.

Timetables can also be used to support people to understand the concept of 'now' and 'next' by displaying activities in a chain and highlighting the current activity and supporting the person to remove the symbol of the completed activity into a 'finished' box.

Visual timetables can be used to support people to increase their understanding of daily routines. They can be linked into the activities that are taking place by detaching objects of reference, symbols or pictures from the timetable and physically taking them to an activity. This makes the contextual link between the timetable and the activities that are taking place. Once an activity is finished, the object, symbol or picture can be returned to the timetable before looking at the next activity.

Timetables can also be a useful tool in supporting people to conceptualise time, for example 'yesterday', 'tomorrow', 'at the end of the week', or even the length of an activity. Depending on the level of understanding of the individual, an arrow or another symbol may be used to indicate the location of the present time on the timetable (for example, which day or session) which can be moved from one location on the timetable to another.

The length of time of an activity can be conveyed, if this is appropriate for the person, by changing the size of the space for each activity. For example, the symbol for lunch might be in a smaller space than 'cookery'.

Think creatively about how visual timetables are presented. For example, activities can be displayed on a mini-whiteboard which can be easily updated regularly, especially when a person needs the reassurance of knowing what is happening now and what is happening next. Timetables can be made to be portable, for example in a book. Consider concertinaed pages, rather than turning pages, as some people may find it difficult to understand or remember a sequence from previous pages. Hinging bookmark-sized cards with a paper fastener at one end to make a fan is a good way to present a sequence of events to someone; this method also has the advantage of being able to reveal parts of the sequence (for example, what is happening now, or next).

Timetables should be tailored to the communication needs of the people who use them. Consider the level of symbolic development of the person or group of people using the timetable. A combination of different media can be used as appropriate, such as symbols, pictures, photographs, objects and words.

The presentation of the timetable should also be considered:

- How much information is presented? For example, a full week, one day or one activity. Are all aspects of the time period included or just key activities?

- How are the timescales represented? For example, days of the week, time, length of activities. Consider whether you need to represent the timescale or if it is enough to provide a 'now and next' type of format.

- How do you indicate the present? For example, today is Wednesday or we are now doing this activity in the sequence.

- How do you communicate that an activity or event has been finished? Consider putting removable symbols in a 'finished' box, using a tick box or covering the symbol.

- How are activities represented? For example, with words, symbols, pictures, photos or objects.

- What layout works for individuals who are using the timetable – is the person able to follow it from left to right or top to bottom? Is a linear timetable more appropriate than a grid? Do you need to link the sections (for example, using an arrow) or is it clearer to simply position the sections next to each other?

© Martin Goodwin, Jennie Miller and Cath Edwards  Speechmark

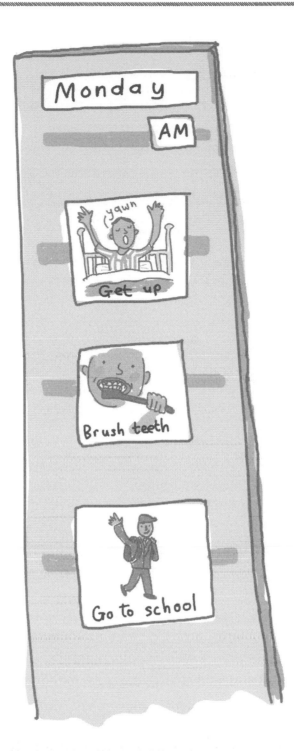

## Reflection

1   Cut round some pictures that are of an equal size.

2   On a piece of A2-sized paper or card, use the pictures to create different layouts for a visual timetable.

3   Consider the differences, benefits and solutions or disadvantages of each layout that was used to make your visual timetable.  How might the different styles suit different people who you know or support?

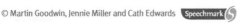

## Examples of good practice

A college supports students to make their own visual timetables at the beginning of each term. These are kept in their diary so that they can be supported to refer to the timetables throughout the day at college. Family or support staff at home use the visual timetables to support the person to communicate about what is going to happen that day at college or what they have been doing during the day.

A youth group has a visual timetable which is used to plan the activities for that session. The board has a set structure which is permanent and the young people choose activities represented by symbols, photographs and words. These are attached to the board in the appropriate sections.

A supported tenancy uses visual timetables to show which support workers are on duty for different shifts. The support workers each have a set of photos of themselves which are attached by Velcro to the appropriate shift. The timetable shows today and tomorrow. Day shifts are indicated by a symbol of a sun, waking night shifts are indicated by symbol of a moon and stars and sleep-in shifts are indicated by a symbol of a bed. Tenants can be supported to look at the timetable to see which support worker will be supporting them.

A leisure centre has made its timetable of activities more accessible by using simple pictures to show which sessions are offered in each time period.

A support worker helps Damien to understand the sequence of events in the morning by making a blank timetable board with Velcro on each section and providing objects of reference which he understands. Damien is given the opportunity to touch and hold each of the objects that represent the activities for the morning and is then helped to place them on his timetable using the Velcro. As the morning progresses, Damien is helped to check what is happening next by touching the relevant object. He is also helped to remove the object which relates to the activity which has just been completed and to place it in his 'finished' box.

Speechmark

# Key-rings

Key-rings are so named because they resemble a key-ring with a selection of small objects or cards ('keys') with pictures or symbols on them, attached by a loop. The advantage of key-rings is that they are a portable communication tool as well as easy and cheap to make. Key-rings can easily be tailored to the communication needs of individuals according to their level of symbolic development. They can also be made up of a combination of small objects, pictures and symbols as required.

Key-rings can work best with a selection of up to about 12 'keys'. Separate key-rings for different themes can be made. These can be grouped into themes and identified by adding a front cover or tag. When using pictures or symbols, key-rings can easily be made durable by printing them on card and laminating them. When laminating, it is best to use matt laminates to avoid reflection and glare. Using text alongside pictures and symbols encourages communication partners to use the same language when supporting people to use the resource.

## Reflection

1   List the benefits and disadvantages of using key-rings to support people with learning disabilities.

2   How could you overcome some of the disadvantages?

When making a key-ring, some aspects to consider include:

- Does it help the person to communicate what they want to say?

- Where the key-ring is kept, so that people can independently access it.

- Are there duplicate copies, so both the communication partner and the person themselves can access them?

- Use things that are motivating to the person, not just commands! Remember, using the key-ring should be a two-way communication process.

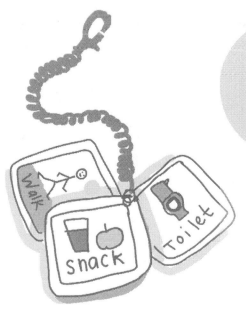

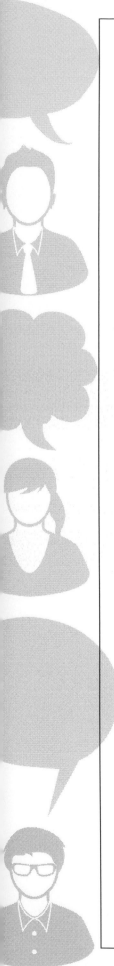

## Examples of good practice

Harry uses limited speech to communicate and people who don't know him find him difficult to understand. He has three key-rings which he made at school. He likes to have them near him and takes them with him in his rucksack whenever he is out. One of the key-rings has 'keys' which communicate:

- I need to go to the toilet (a symbol of a toilet)

- I am thirsty (symbols of a coffee cup with steam rising and a separate key showing a glass)

- I am hungry (a few keys with symbols for sweets, crisps and a meal on them, and a laminated chocolate wrapper – Harry's favourite)

- I am cold (a cartoon character of a cold person)

- I am too hot (a cartoon character of a hot person)

- I want to go home now (a symbol of a house)

- It is too noisy – I need to go somewhere quiet (a cartoon character with his hands over his ears).

Another key-ring has a series of activities that Harry likes to do, including:

- going to the park (a simple line drawing of a swing and a slide)

- drawing (a drawing in crayon that Harry has done for the key-ring)

- painting (a painting that Harry has done for the key-ring)

- craft (a small laminated collage)

- music (a picture of some musical instruments that Harry likes to use)

- listening to music (a photo of Harry with his headphones on)

- watching TV (a symbol of a television)

- quiet time (a cartoon character with his hands over his ears).

Each key has some text on it reinforcing what Harry is communicating.

Claire is a community support worker who supports people to go out for short sessions. She uses key-rings to support people to choose what they want to do at the beginning of each session. Claire made the resources herself by collecting pictures and symbols and taking photographs of activities that were available to do in the area. Before each session, Claire chooses a selection of

'keys' according to activities that are open, the weather, the time available and what she knows the person enjoys doing. The appropriate bookmark-sized keys are fastened using
a paper fastener at one end. The keys can be displayed all together or one at a time, as appropriate, to support people to make choices about the activities that are available.

A school uses sets of key-rings with keys that are relevant to specific activities. For example, in the cookery classroom, there are two sets of key-rings, one with instructions on them (including washing hands, putting an apron on, mixing and pouring) and one set with different utensils on (including a bowl, spoon and rolling-pin). There are several copies of each key-ring. Some are made up of symbols, some with pictures and some with objects of reference. As the class completes the activity, the classroom assistants use the appropriate key-rings, according to the person's symbol development, to support them to follow instructions and find the items they need.

# Objects of reference

The term 'objects of reference' was first used by Jan van Dijk in the 1960s to describe the use of objects as a communication tool with people who were deaf-blind. They are also sometimes called 'signifiers'. The approach is now also used with people with learning disabilities as their main method of communication or to reinforce other methods of communication. Objects are concrete, as opposed to abstract (see 'Development of communication' section), and are one of the simplest forms of communication because they are most similar to what they represent.

Attaching meaning to the actual object is the earliest stage of symbol development. This is achieved through association in routines and cause and effect. For example, pyjamas represent going to bed, a book represents sitting down for story time, a cup or glass represents a drink. Over time, the object stands for something more than itself and comes to represent what is likely to happen next. For example, putting a coat on can mean 'we are going out'; sitting at the table with a plate and knife and fork can mean 'we are going to eat a meal'. Later, objects can be used to influence what is going to happen. For example, 'If I give Granddad a book, he reads it to me': the book is no longer just a book; it represents a request; for Granddad to read a story. The objects can also be used to facilitate choice and simple decision-making: for example, 'Granddad might show me three books; if I take that one, that is the one he reads'.

Supporting people to use objects to communicate follows the same process, beginning with reinforcing the association between an object and what it represents. This is achieved through repetition: for example, always giving the person an arm band before leaving the house to go swimming, talking about swimming while holding the arm band on the journey, using the arm band during swimming, then holding the arm band when talking about swimming afterwards. Over a period of time, a part of the arm band may be used or associations may be developed between the object and a picture or symbol of the arm band to aid further symbolic development.

Supporting people to make the association between objects and what they can represent enables people to:

- focus attention while talking about the related subject or activity
- understand what is about to happen
- make choices between two or more things
- make requests
- develop skills towards using more abstract and complex representations such as symbols, pictures and signs.

Speechmark

The objects chosen to support someone should reflect that person's ability and interests. The object may be something that is actually used in that activity or it may be something more abstract to what it represents (eg a toy car to represent going out in the car) or something chosen by the individual even if this may appear completely unrelated (eg a piece of cloth to represent having quiet time to rest or sleep). Often, observing people's routines and how they do things will reveal an object that has significance to that person for an activity.

Objects tend to represent an activity but they can also represent people, events and ideas. For example:

- a wooden spoon represents cooking
- a CD represents music
- a small plastic plate represents meal times
- an empty fries box from a well-known fast food restaurant represents going there for a meal
- a purse could represent 'going to the shops'
- some shoelaces might represent a walking group
- a pair of knitting needles might represent Granny.

When introducing objects of reference, it is important to consider what the object represents. Does the person already have an object that they associate with that activity? the object should be easy to find, portable and easily replaced (in case it goes missing or gets damaged). In view of health and safety, it is important to consider whether the object poses any hazards with regard to mouthing, swallowing or choking.

More than one object can be used to build up meanings: for example, 'going swimming with school' might be an arm band and a small part of the school uniform.

Objects of reference should be available to the person. They can be kept:

- in a box
- hung on hooks
- in a bag
- on a wheelchair tray
- attached to a timetable
- attached by Velcro to a door (to reinforce an activity, eg a plate on the dining hall door, a small book on the library door).

It is important that the people supporting the person also understand what the object of reference means; otherwise, the object may not support communication as intended and can lead to misunderstandings, confusion and frustration by both parties. This information can be recorded in care plans, a communication dictionary and/or in a laminated book kept with the objects. These will need to be updated and modified as objects or meanings change.

## Reflection

1 Consider what objects you would use to communicate the following to people with learning disabilities:

- toilet

- cooking

- time to go to sleep

- play time.

2 Consider how objects of reference could be introduced and used with someone you know.

In addition to objects which are tactile and visual, other stimuli may be provided to make reference to events, places or daily routines. Consider how you might use smell, taste or sounds as well as touch and sight, particularly for people with complex needs. This is called *sensory referencing*. Sensory referencing can be used collaboratively or singularly to represent contexts, events, locations or people. Smell is a particularly powerful sense and is a useful tool for people with more complex needs. Examples of olfactory (smell) stimuli that can be used may include spices or herbs for cooking or a gardening activity, scented candles which are used at bath time, chlorine on a swimming costume which reminds a person of swimming. However, care must be taken with using smells for referencing because they tend to persist and to spread beyond the area where they are relevant.

Consider how you can support people to develop their communication skills from using objects of reference to other methods of communication. Using objects of reference alongside other methods bridges the two methods and supports understanding by helping a person to associate the new method of communication with the object and the meaning. Eventually, the original object is no longer required as the person associates the new method of communication with the meaning. A person's transition to the next stage of development will vary. Some people will progress in really small steps and others will make more significant progress.

Supporting people to develop their communication skills from using objects of reference may be achieved in small steps in the following ways:

- mounting part of the object on a board, for example half a tennis ball or half a plastic cup

- mounting a symbol on chunky foam cut in the shape of the symbol to give it a tactile element, for example the shape of a cup

- using string to add tactile definition to the outline of a symbol.

## Examples of good practice

A school attaches objects of reference to doors to support children to learn the function of rooms. These objects correspond to the objects of reference that are used with some children on their visual timetable.

Lizzie hated using the accessible transport because, for a time, she hated going to school. After the issues with school were resolved, Lizzie still hated getting on the transport, even if she was not going to school. Staff on the transport suggested to Mum and Dad that Lizzie might benefit from using objects of reference that she could hold on the bus which represented where she was going or what she would be doing. Mum and Dad put a bag of items together. When Lizzie was going to meet her sister to go shopping at the weekend, she would hold a bag she only used for the occasion; when she was doing cooking, her favourite class at school, she would hold a wooden spoon during the journey, and so on. Mum and Dad, the staff on the transport and the staff at her destination all handled the object with Lizzie when talking about or doing the activity that the object represented. After only a few weeks, Lizzie's anxiety reduced significantly when using the accessible transport. Those who knew her well also noticed that she would choose certain objects out of her bag to show them; these represented her favourite activities. Lizzie was using the objects of reference to show preference.

Melissa loved to use the sensory room at her day service. She associated the sensory room with the essential oils that were used during the session. When considering the objects of reference that would be meaningful to Melissa for the activities that she enjoyed the support staff used a small bottle of lavender oil.

A nature centre which was used regularly by a local school that supported people with a learning disability put together a box of tactile objects representing different activities that they offered. A piece of bark mounted on a board was used to represent the woodland walk, a fishing net represented pond dipping, a large goose feather represented feeding the ducks and a small pair of binoculars was used to represent going birdwatching.

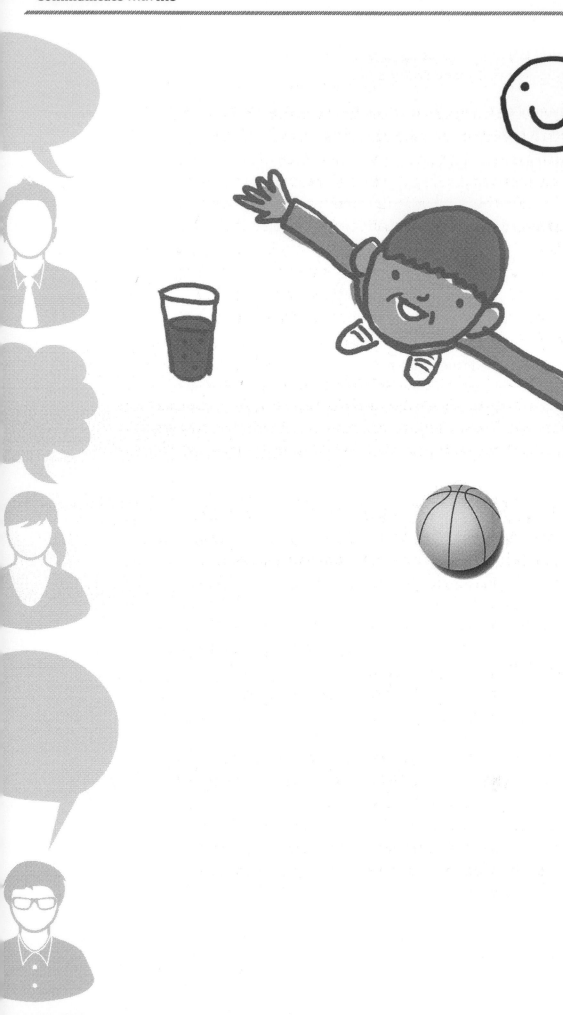

Speechmark

# Using technology

There have been enormous advances in the use of computer technology to support people to communicate. Communication aids that use any form of computer technology are defined as low mid and high-tech aids. There is not always a consensus on the definition of these categories; however, they are all electronic and use computer technology. Generally, the more technologically advanced an aid is, the higher the category is. Low-tech aids include simple switches such as BIGmack™ and Gotalk4™ which play pre-recorded or synthesised verbal messages which are accessed by pressing a button or symbol. More high-tech options such as VOCAs (voice output communication aids) often require more input or allow the user to navigate more pages, offering increased choice. Higher-tech products can be programmed to grow and develop to meet individual needs.

It is important that communication aids use vocabulary that the person would want to use and can expand as their communication and lifestyle develops. Technological aids can be augmentative (in addition to other communication systems or speech) or alternative (used instead of speech). Communication aids differ greatly depending on their purpose.

For the effective use of technological communication aids, the person using them needs to have an understanding of cause and effect ('when I do this, that happens'). The choice of communication aid should be appropriate to a person's cognitive and physical ability as well as their level of communication.

A first stage in supporting people to understand the process of communication using technology is to ensure that the technology is motivating and pleasurable to the person, such as operating a toy with a switch or a switch-operated music system. This helps the person to understand a basic function of communication in that they can make basic needs and wants known.

A range of communication devices can be used depending on the person's communication development and cognitive ability. This may start with presenting people with a single option device with one meaning, to selecting a desired outcome from a range of options presented to a person in a choice board format. Other aids can facilitate the communication of more complex concepts and functions of communication by enabling the expression of, for example, sentences, ideas, observations and conversation.

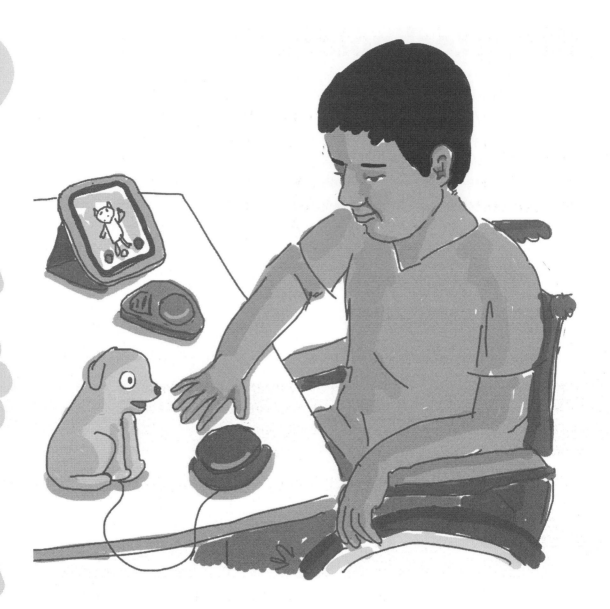

Technological aids can be products that have either been designed exclusively for the purpose of supporting communication or use existing technology such as a personal computer which has been adapted for use as a communication tool.

The continued advances in the technology that are readily available to us, such as touch-screen phones, tablets and all their applications, will make such aids more easily tailored to meet individual need and become more affordable. A range of applications and software exist to develop communication and interaction and are available from app stores and specialist websites (see 'Further reading which resources').

Some technological aids can be expensive to purchase but there are resource libraries available where aids can be borrowed for a small fee or free of charge. Sometimes aids can be tried before purchasing. Specialist advice is available from speech and language therapists and AAC (augmentative and alternative communication) specialists.

Speechmark

## Reflection

1 It is easy to find out about the technology that is available. Try entering terms such as 'augmentative alternative communication' into a browser on the internet or look at some of the suggested websites in the further reading section at the end of this book.

2 Consider the people who you support or know. How could technology facilitate their ability to communicate?

### Examples of good practice

The BIGmack offers a single message facility when a button is pressed. This is a good tool for teaching simple 'cause and effect' and can help users to start to initiate communication.

John is a child with profound and multiple disabilities who needs support with feeding because of his physical disability. John's support staff noticed that he was not enjoying meal times. He showed this by rejecting the food that was offered and some staff thought that John felt rushed at times. A BIGmack was programmed with the word 'more' (a concept that John was beginning to understand) to offer him more control at meal times. John was then taught to press the BIGmack switch when he was ready for his food. This was achieved by teaching him to associate the use of the BIGmack with his request for more in the following way. When John was asked if he was 'ready for more' and he was observed through non-verbal communication, to say he wanted more, John's support staff prompted him to press the BIGmack switch with his hand under their hand. This taught him to learn to associate his non-verbal request for 'more' with the action of pressing the switch, which in turn verbalised the word 'more'. After a few weeks of using 'more' on the BIGmack, John could control when he wanted food. Teaching 'cause and effect' can be promoted through a variety of fun toys which can be adapted or purchased to promote communication and play.

Switches can be used to operate a wide variety of equipment to support and enable inclusion.

There are a range of products available that can support communication using simple touch-responsive technology. These show a personal message that can be used if a person gets lost and a talking photo album so that a person can explain what the pictures are about using pre-recorded messages.

 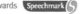

Other examples have more complex ways of requesting and communicating through the use of concept boards. As the person's understanding of how to use technology grows, and they learn concepts such as categorising, prepositions and early language skills, they may be able to move on to more complex aids such as VOCA (voice output communication aids), for example Dynavox™ or Orac™.

Computers and tablets are becoming increasingly affordable and offer a range of innovative communication aids and interactive software to engage people.

Speechmark

# Communicating using signs

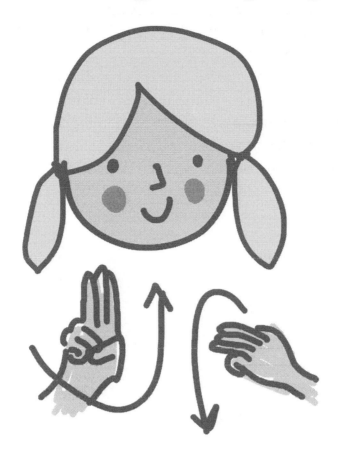

There are three main signing systems used in the UK.

British Sign Language was officially recognised as a language in its own right in 2003. It is not dependent on spoken English and has a separate grammatical structure and syntax. It uses finger spelling and signs alongside gestures, facial expressions and body language. There is also a deaf-blind tactile alphabet used by people with dual sensory loss which is based on deaf manual signs.

Makaton™ is a language programme using signs and symbols (see the section on page 125) to help people to communicate. It is designed to support spoken language and the signs and symbols are used with speech, in spoken word order. Makaton was originally developed by Margaret Walker, Katherine Johnston and Tony Comforth in the 1970s and it continues to be developed by The Makaton Charity (www.makaton.org). In the UK it is based on British Sign Language: each adaptation is based on native sign language to be culturally acceptable. Makaton is the only sign or symbol programme with evidence-based research supporting its effectiveness.

Makaton has a core vocabulary of around 450 words or concepts which are grouped into stages supporting language development. This vocabulary of signs and symbols can be built up to form phrases and sentences; Makaton can support full literacy. There is also a 'resource' vocabulary which has over 11,000 concepts covering a variety of topics including transport, animals, food, people, personal health, and so on.

Signalong is a sign-supporting system that is also based on British Sign Language and loosely modelled on the structure of the Derbyshire Language Scheme. It was initially developed by a school for children with learning disability in Kent in 1992. One sign is used per concept and signs are used in spoken word order. Signalong now includes over 15,000 published signs and is considered by them as the signing system of choice for workers in autism and for Total Communication applications.

The main differences between the two systems are that Signalong is a system for signs only but Makaton also provides a resource of symbols to support written language. Makaton is structured into developmental stages, whereas Signalong is built up according to individual need and use.

Another important signing system is tactile-based sign. This is sometimes referred to as hands-on, co-active or body signing. This approach uses adapted signs that are physically made on (agreed) parts of the body or a communication partner moulds the person's hands into the appropriate signs to communicate with them. Tactile signing is primarily used with people with multiple sensory impairments and people who are deaf-blind but may be used with people with profound and multiple learning disabilities if it is meaningful and they understand. It is important to consider the person's level of symbolic development.

When signing, it is important to remember:

- Sign alongside speech, not instead of speech. Both are an aid to supporting the development of speech.

- Sign in time with words; this will also help you to concentrate on key words and make your speech simpler.

- Use signing as part of a Total Communication approach; remember to use facial expression, body language and tone of voice as well as speech to accompany signs.

- You can use signs (as appropriate) even if the person does not communicate.

- Be clear and consistent with signs.

- Consider people's ability. Not everybody will be able to use signs due to motor coordination or processing difficulties. Some people will find it difficult to simultaneously understand speech and follow signing.

- When people use their own signs or adapt them, make sure you are aware of this. Don't discourage people from using their own signs – recognise what they are signing but continue to model the correct sign.

- Record signs that are recognised by the person and those that are used by them (in care plans, a communication dictionary, etc).

If someone uses a sign-supporting system or symbols, it is really important for everybody who supports that person to understand and use the same system. People supporting the individual need to receive training and regularly practise vocabulary to maintain knowledge and consistency.

## Reflection

1  Learn how to introduce yourself and sign your name using finger spelling.

2  Set yourself a challenge to learn five simple signs that you might use with people you meet.

## Examples of good practice

Ali has some verbal communication skills. He uses sign at school alongside any songs that are sung in music groups and at story time. All of the teachers at school use sign to support all verbal communication with the children. Although Ali doesn't use many signs himself, his teacher has noticed that his understanding of activities in the classroom, aspects of school routine and his overall understanding of verbal communication have increased. When the youth group he attends on a Friday night also started using sign when referring to activities and routines, Ali became more settled and involved.

When Naomi moved into a supported tenancy from children's services, her staff team arranged training from the Total Communication Therapist at the college she attended, so that her support team could learn the signs and symbols that Naomi used. Although Naomi had some verbal communication,

 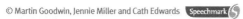

her understanding and ability to communicate how she felt was increased when the staff team also used signs to communicate verbally with her. This was hugely beneficial in supporting Naomi to settle into her new home and to adjust to the new environment and routines. It also helped her to express how she was feeling so that she could be supported more effectively through the transition.

Collin has profound and multiple learning disabilities and visual impairment. He would become afraid when some people suddenly spoke to him because he could not always see them approaching. Collin's support worker introduced a system where staff and visitors were asked to approach Collin slowly from in front and to gently take his thumb to indicate 'Hello' before starting to talk to him. Over time, Collin was no longer startled when people initiated conversation with him.

Speechmark

# Independence boards or sheets

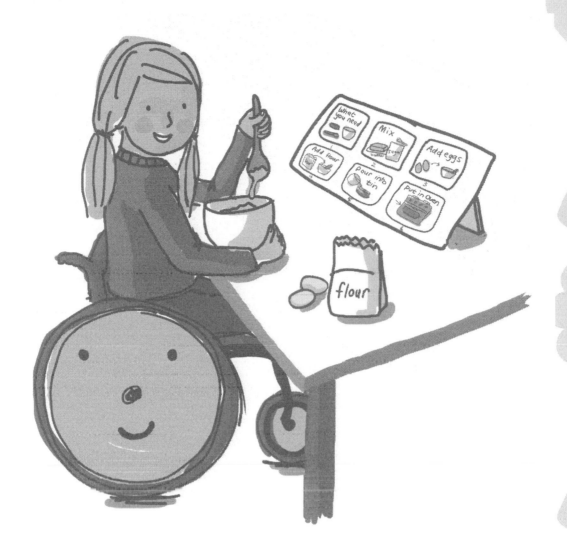

Independence boards, or independence sheets, support a person to become more independent by splitting a task or an activity into a series of simple steps. The instructions may support the completion of a task or an activity in the correct order. The independence boards use symbols, pictures or objects (laid out in order or in boxes) and usually also include easy words.

One example is the process of making toast. This activity involves getting the bread out of the bag; putting it in the toaster, pressing the button down, getting a plate, knife and butter out ready for the toast; waiting until the toast pops up, and spreading butter on the toast. The toast is then ready to eat. The person may be able to do each of these tasks independently of each other; however, to chain the sequence of actions together so that they flow naturally is a different skill altogether. The accessible independence board is a valuable tool to use alongside verbal prompts. It is also particularly useful when supporting someone to rely less on step-by-step verbal support.

When making information easy to understand, it is important to use symbols or pictures that a person understands. What is accessible for one person is not necessarily accessible to another. When producing resources, it is not always possible to tailor-make information for each individual. However, information can be prepared using a range of different formats such as pictures, symbols and words for each piece of information, so that it can be used for several individuals or in a group situation where people have different abilities.

Independence boards can be fixed resources which outline a set sequence. They can also be a template to support someone to sequence an activity by attaching symbols or pictures on the board in order.

Be creative about the use of independence boards. For example, consider using them for shopping lists, which might use pictures, symbols or real wrappers or packaging for items on the list, lists or learning how to use technology such as selecting a television channel.

## Reflection

1 Consider how you could use independence boards with the people you support.

2 Think of an activity. List the stages or separate elements of the activity in order and consider how you would represent the instructions for each element using different methods of communication. Consider how you would support someone to understand and follow the process.

## Examples of good practice

A youth group used an independence board to support young people to print their own design on a T-shirt. Using this method helped the group to stay focused on each part of the process and involved them in talking about each stage before it was done. As well as their T-shirt, each young person had a copy of the process to take home. This created opportunities to talk with family, friends and support staff about what they had done.

When planning to go on holiday, Julie was supported to list what she needed to do to prepare. Julie and her support worker talked about what needed to be done. Julie then drew a picture for each task and her support worker wrote underneath it. Julie liked to choose in which order she completed tasks and ticked off each one when it was done.

Speechmark

At home, Farahat is supported to make her packed lunch more independently. On the work top, she has a laminated spiral-bound book on a stand. She can use the pictures to follow the stages independently – each sheet has pictures in a flow diagram for one stage of making her lunch. Once each stage is complete, she turns the page to reveal the next stage in the sequence. The last page is a big picture of a lunch box with all the things in it she needs, so that she can check she has not missed anything.

Paul's mother helped him to find items on his shopping trip by placing real wrappers and packaging on a shopping list for him to find, in the order that he would come to them when walking round the shop.

# Documenting communication

When working closely with someone, a knowledge base is built up about that person, including how they communicate. This will include information such as a person's preferred methods of communication, their level of symbolic development, the specific signs or symbols they use, and how they communicate specific things such as pain.

It may take a lot of time and experience for practitioners to understand how a person communicates and how best to communicate with them. It is very important to record this knowledge to maintain continuity of support for people. When information about how people communicate is not recorded or shared, this may result in them becoming further disabled and, in some cases, not having their basic health and support needs met. However, it is important to state that while the process of documenting communication is beneficial, documents should not be used as a replacement for talking to people and checking with them about how they communicate or, indeed, any wishes they may have.

Effectively documenting people's communication provides a way of promoting consistency between practitioners, and helps new practitioners to quickly gain a shared understanding of how to support someone. Furthermore, collating information and reviewing existing documents creates an opportunity for people to share experiences and knowledge about supporting an individual, thereby enhancing each other's understanding of that person and how best to support them.

Documents that record how a person communicates should be tailored to the individual. There are a range of methods that have been developed to effectively record communication, including sections in Sally Millar's 'Communication Passports' and Helen Sanderson's 'Communication Dictionaries' (see the links in 'Further reading and resources'). Some services have their own pro formas in place which can be adapted to meet individual needs. Be creative about how you document communication. Consider recording a DVD, taking photographs or making a poster.

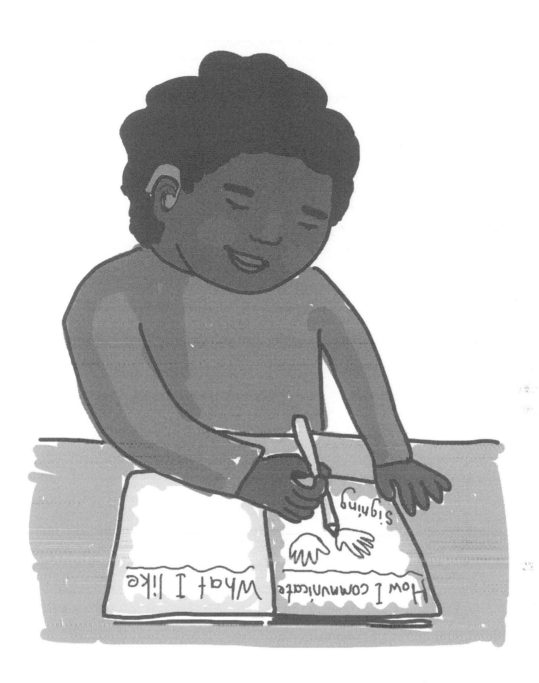

Below are some examples of aspects of communication that may be included:

- emotions (happiness, sadness, enjoyment, excitement, anxiety, frustration, etc)

- pain, discomfort, feeling unwell

- feeling too hot or too cold

- whether they are hungry or thirsty

- that they like or dislike something

- that they want to do another activity, go home, use the toilet, and so on

- how they can be supported to make choices.

The record should include the methods of communication that the person uses:

- signs that are used and those that are recognised

- objects of reference used, when these are used, and supporting information to new people about how to use them

- pictures and symbols the person recognises and uses

- whether they have key-rings, communication boards, high-tech aids, etc

- their level of understanding of speech and ability to express themselves verbally.

General pointers to aid good communication should also be included, such as:

- I can't hear well if there is a lot of background noise; I lip-read a little so please don't cover your mouth or turn away when talking to me

- Jo appears to understand a lot, however it is important to check comprehension with discreet questions so that, if she doesn't fully understand, you can explain in another way

- Rhiannon needs to take her time when thinking so allow time for her to respond

- Even though David doesn't sign himself, when other people sign, this increases his understanding of what other people are saying.

When collecting information, or reviewing documents, it is important to involve the individual and those who know them best. Spending time discussing how people communicate and how they are supported promotes continuity in support and builds on everybody's understanding of the person. Family, friends and other professionals may see the person in different environments and may be able to draw from a knowledge spanning many years.

## Reflection

1   What are the benefits of documenting communication methods?

2   Can you think of any disadvantages of documenting communication?

3   List some creative ways in which you could document information to make it accessible and meaningful to people with whom you work.

## Examples of good practice

Ibrahim communicates using a lot of facial expressions. It takes time to learn what his facial vocabulary means, so his carers took pictures and made a short DVD. In this way other people supporting him could more quickly understand what his different facial expressions meant.

At home, Pete's support staff know him very well. They have supported him to make a range of symbol key-rings which he uses at home, with his Community Support Worker and when he stays with his family. Pete's staff team have also put together a document over time. Included in this is a section where each page is divided into three columns which are headed 'When Pete does this ...' (eg shouts 'Awhooooooo oh oh oh' while rocking back and forwards on his feet), 'We think this means ...' (Pete is happy and enjoying himself), 'And we respond by ...' (echoing what he is saying with him). The book was put together by his staff team at home, his Community Support Worker and his mother. When Pete started at a new day service, the staff team copied the document for them so that they could use it to learn how Pete communicates.

A day service has a pro forma that it uses as part of the referral process. They have designed a section to capture information from people who know the person well, such as family or other support staff. The section asks specific questions around communication such as how the person can be best supported to make choices and how they express pain and discomfort. There is also a list of different methods of communication to indicate how people communicate and to give an indication of their level of symbol development. This information forms the basis of plans when
as the person starts the service and is added to as support staff get to know the person themselves.

# Reflecting diversity

When preparing or purchasing communication resources, it is important to consider how these represent our diverse communities in relation, for example, to ethnicity, faith, culture, gender, sexuality, age and disability.

It is important that people identify with and relate to the resources that are used to support communication. People need to develop a secure and positive sense of their own identity. A person's background and individuality will be the most significant source of that identity. It is important that people can see themselves, their family and familiar experiences reflected in the resources that they use. If the picture or symbol looks different, some people with learning disabilities may not be able to identify with the person who they are seeing in the picture or symbol. If a resource is tailored to the individual and is about them (for example, using a story to explore their social situation), there may be a need to use pictures or symbols of the same gender, skin colour or even hair colour.

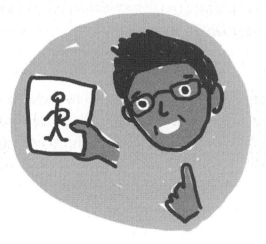

The communication resources that are available should reflect who a person is and what is important to them. Resources should inspire and motivate the person to communicate and provide a method of expression about their life and what is important to them, so that they can make choices and communicate in ways that are relevant.

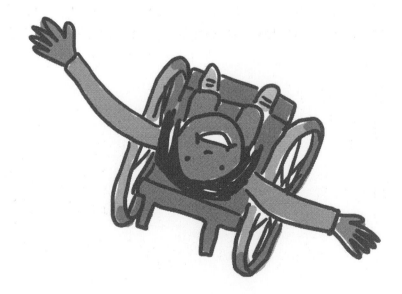

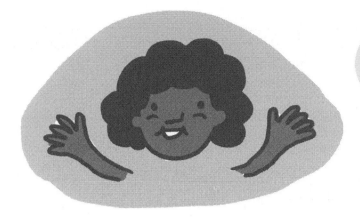

Communication resources that are limited to stereotypical activities that always show the same type of person don't always facilitate this and may even be a barrier to communication.

Where communication resources are shared or relate to people other than an individual, these should include culturally representative images and different aspects of life, so that diverse communities and people are promoted and valued. There is always diversity in communities, even if this is not reflected in the people who access a provision.

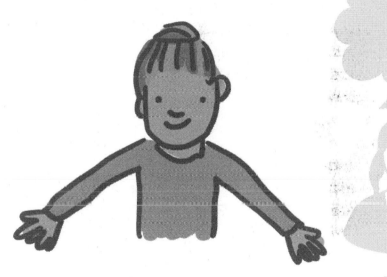

It is good practice to review the messages that are given by the resources that are used within services – from key-rings and choice boards used by individuals to photos and videos which are used to make a website accessible. By carefully selecting resources that reflect the diversity of the people who are supported within the provision, and the communities that the provision is part of, inclusion and positive values can be promoted.

Shared culture and the diversity of communities, as well as the diversity of the nation as a whole, can be communicated through events and aspects of daily life such as:

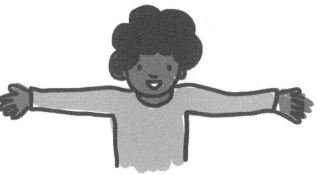

- different faith celebrations, eg Christmas, Easter, Chinese New Year, Passover, Eid, Diwali

- various dress styles – reflected in pictures or photographs

- a range of ages – some communication resources are

designed for use with children, so it is mportant to consider how teenagers and adults may feel using them

- different ethnic groups reflected in pictures or photographs

- variety in food and drink

- representation of disabled and non-disabled people and different disabilities

- different languages

- a variety of music or art forms.

## Reflection

Consider your community and/or the one in which your service or setting is located.

1 Why is it important to reflect diversity within services?

2 How is the diversity of the community reflected within the service or setting?

3 How are different events or aspects of daily life represented?

4 What changes would you make to more effectively reflect diversity within the service or setting?

## Examples of good practice

Accessible reading material available to students in a college is accompanied by pictures of adults rather than of children.

Projects at a day service reflect different festivals throughout the year. Supporting communication resources have been made for these.

Nadia's key-ring shows pictures of family members in traditional Egyptian dress. One of the keys allows her to tell people that she is fasting at the moment. On the back of the key, information for staff at the day centre reminds them what she can eat and drink and when. The supporting text is in English and Arabic.

The resource library of a service that supports people in a residential setting has a range of social stories to support people to think about issues such as moving house, experiencing loss and attending funeral services for a range of faiths; transition to a new school; and going on holiday. These depict people of different ethnicities and with different disabilities.

The website for a community support organisation shows pictures of service users with different disabilities, from different ethnic backgrounds and representing a range of ages.

# Tailoring communication methods

People with learning disabilities communicate using diverse communication methods. The way a person communicates is as individual as the person themselves, drawing from a wide range of methods which may include speech, gestures, symbols and signs. These methods may be conventional in that they are recognisable and transferrable, ie words used in the conventional sense with conventional meanings, or signs from British Sign Language or Makaton. Communication methods may also be unconventional or individualised: for example, words or phrases that differ from their literal meaning or signs which are simplified or created by the individual.

When supporting communication, it is important to understand how someone communicates as well as how to respond using a range of communication methods, ensuring that every effort is made to interact and engage.

Achieving good communication is about getting to know the individual, learning about their ways of communicating and then ensuring that their preferred methods are used at every opportunity.

See the sections 'Enabling effective communication' and 'Total Communication' for more information.

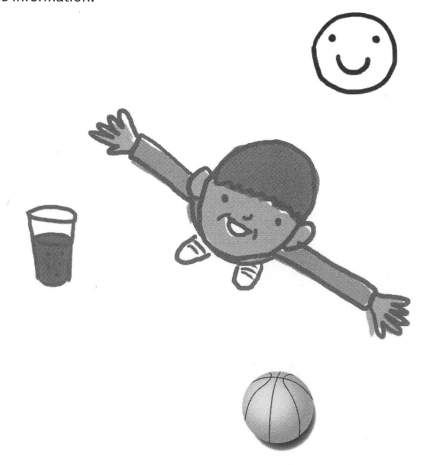

# Service user guide

A service user guide is an introduction to a service and what it offers. It is designed to be used by the people who access that service. It is important that people with learning disabilities have information about the service they use so that they know who people are, how people around them can support them and the facilities or support that is offered by the service. As well as providing information for current service users, a service user guide can provide information for people who want to find out about a service before accessing it.

An accessible service user guide also provides an opportunity to communicate to service users what their rights and responsibilities are, what to do if, for example, they are not happy with an aspect of the service, if they don't feel safe, or what information may be held about them. The guide may also include the views of people who access the service.

Be creative about the format of the guide. Consider making a booklet or portfolio, a DVD, an audio CD or a website.

It follows therefore that the service user guide is accessible to the target audience.

Some aspects to consider might include:

- The communication needs of the people who will be accessing the guide.

- How to make it accessible to a wide range of ability levels or communication preferences without making the document confusing.

- Whether the guide will be made in one format or several different versions (eg using easy words, print with pictures and/or symbols, an audio version, or an audio-visual version).

- The format of the service user guide (eg booklet, DVD, portfolio, web-based).

- Whether aspects of the guide, such as making a complaint or service user responsibilities, could also be delivered through other methods of communication such as drama or workshops.

When making an accessible service user guide, it is important to consult and involve current service users and to include information that is important to them about the service. Being involved in putting together a service user guide creates an opportunity for a group of people to become more aware of the service they use and to explore and reflect on aspects of the service that are important to them.

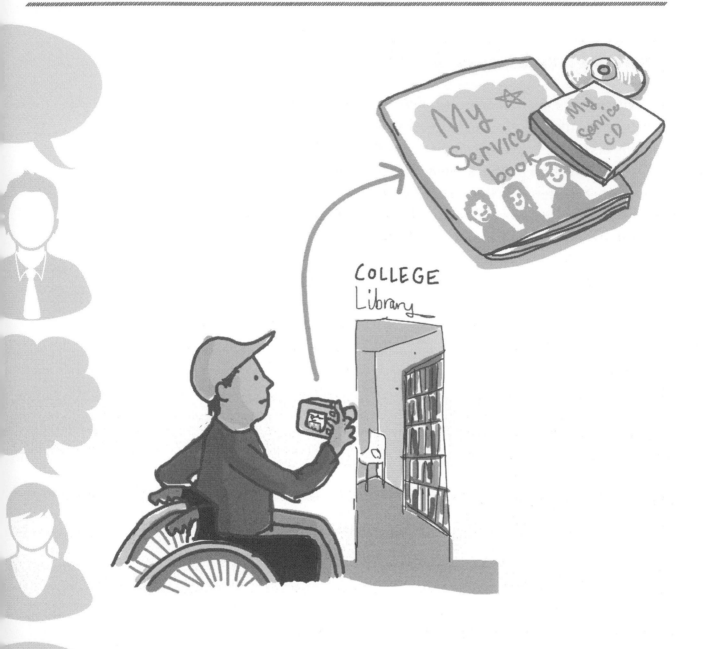

## Reflection

1 What information is currently available to new or potential service users accessing the service you work for?

2 Consider what you would like to know about your service if you were new or considering accessing your service.

Speechmark

## Examples of good practice

A college supported students to create a service user guide which would inform new or potential students about what it was like to attend the college. It included introductions to key staff, information about the facilities available, an introduction to a few current students and what they enjoy doing at college and also some rules and responsibilities. The guide was produced as a DVD ,accompanied by a person signing Makaton™, and as a paper version made accessible through using Widget™ literacy symbols, pictures and easy language. Both are available on the website and are sent out to new students or can be requested by potential students.

A community support service produces a service user guide that is also a guide to activities and opportunities available in the area. The guide is updated by a different group of service users each year. It is available to people as a DVD and on the service website. The guide has a menu of different sections:

- About the service – informing service users of the different options of support available, such as purchasing one-to-one support or purchasing support for two or more friends who want to do the same thing; joining an existing interest group and booking on day trips. Each member of the group involved in writing the guide shows how they use the service and what they enjoy.

- Using the service – including information such as 'What can you expect from staff supporting you?', 'Some guidelines that service users need to follow', 'How to contact the office', 'What to do if you need to cancel support through holiday or illness', 'What to do if you are not happy about something', 'How to increase, decrease, change or cancel hours', and so on.

- What is available to do in the area – a bank of short films showing different activities and opportunities. This is updated and added to each year as required.

A supported employment service supports people with learning disabilities to understand about the different types of work that they can choose to take part in by giving them a talking photo album. This has pictures of the different jobs that they can do and basic information about each job. The person presses a button to listen to the information.

# Making service and events publicity accessible

Making information accessible demonstrates that a service respects and values the people they support. The target audience for publicity tends to be the social worker, carer or family member rather than the individual who will be accessing the service. Making the same information accessible to potential or existing service users creates opportunities for people with learning disabilities to be involved in purchasing services or support and accessing activities and events.

In addition to it being morally right, making information accessible is a legal requirement. In the UK, the Equality Act 2010 consolidated several Acts around discrimination, including the Disability Discrimination Act 1995. It obligates organisations and services to:

- provide (employees and) service users with disabilities with information in an alternative or accessible format

- not leave (employees and) service users with disabilities at a disadvantage.

The Disability Equality Duty 2006 also outlines the legal duty of public sector organisations to promote equality of opportunity for disabled people, which includes making information accessible to them.

Service and events publicity may target new or existing service users and could include information about:

- the services offered

- new activities or opportunities

- open days

- seasonal fairs

- fund-raising events

- information or awareness events for service users

- meetings or consultation events for service users.

When making service and events publicity accessible, consider using more imaginative formats to reach people such as:

- DVDs which are visual and could incorporate signing

- posters, leaflets, letters and newsletters which could be made accessible using pictures, symbols, cartoons and simple words

- providing information around service and events publicity as part of the service's website.

## Reflection

1 Create a draft poster to advertise your service or an event (the information needs to be short, to the point and easy to understand for the people with whom you work).

2 Consider the advantages or disadvantages of your design.

## Examples of good practice

Newsletters are a great way to regularly publicise and promote activities and events within a service. A service that supports adults with learning disabilities within supported tenancies helped a group of service users to manage the production of a newsletter. Members of the team were supported to carry out all the tasks, including gathering information, putting the newsletter together, making the information accessible, taking photographs for articles or future events and distributing the finished product. The practitioners who supported the service user team all received training around making information accessible. The newsletter began to be shaped by suggestions made by team members. In addition to publicising events and opportunities within the service, it had a section devoted to birthday and celebration messages, articles and details about other services accessed by tenants and a section for selling or giving away items such as furniture and crockery within the tenancies.

To advertise the services provided by a local advocacy service, the organisation designed and printed posters using simple cartoons to illustrate different aspects of the service they offered. The posters were distributed around local day services, youth groups, children's homes, supported tenancies, schools and colleges for people with a learning disability.

A new project to promote art in the community was set up, run by a community support group for people with learning disabilities. The leaflets and posters that were used to promote the project were made accessible using simple words and clear accessible graphics. These were distributed to colleges, day services, local community resources such as the library, and cafés, as well as to service managers for local services to distribute.

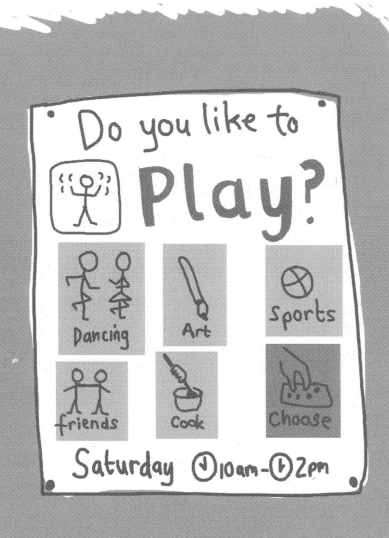

# Making websites accessible

Making websites easy to understand is an important way of respecting the rights of people to access information in ways they can understand. It also respects their right not to be excluded from opportunities that other people have. Companies and services are now required by law to provide equal access to information and services. It is against the law to treat a disabled person 'less favourably' than non-disabled people.

In the UK, Section III of the Disability Discrimination Act 1995, which refers to accessible websites, came into force in 1999 and the Code of Practice for this section of the Disability Discrimination Act was published in 2002. These requirements are now incorporated in the Disability Equality Act 2010.

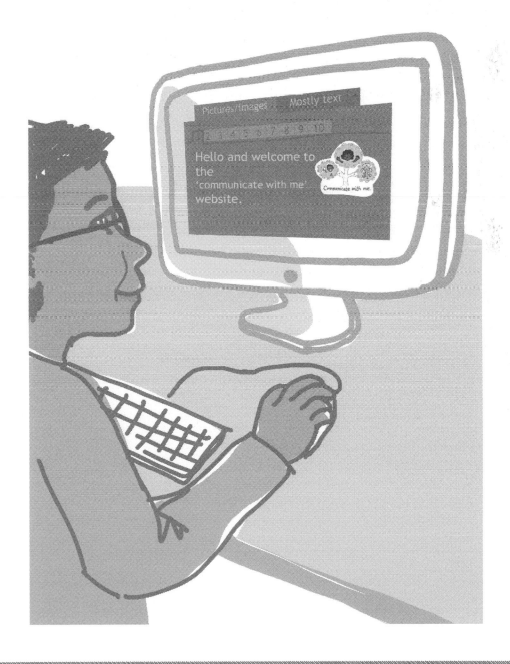

The World Wide Web Consortium (W3C) was set up in the mid-nineties to develop a set of international standards for the World Wide Web which was designed to promote compatibility and consistency between web pages. The Web Accessibility Initiative (WAI), which is part of the W3C, promotes guidelines and techniques in making sites accessible; these are considered to be the international standard for web accessibility.

Ability to access a website includes how people perceive, understand, navigate and interact with the site. The starting point for designing an accessible website should be to consult with service users, families and carers to establish the requirements of a site and what people already find useful on other sites. The same group should be involved in testing and giving feedback throughout the process. It is important to consider software that people may use to make information accessible such as 'Read Aloud', which reads text, and Widgit 'Point', which converts words into symbols, where the user hovers the mouse over the word. It is also important to ensure that websites are compatible with these tools.

It is not essential to be an expert in web design when commissioning a site. However, it is important to be aware of the different methods available whereby people can be supported to access information within a site. Below are a few links for further information.

- W3C quick tips to make accessible websites: www.w3.org/WAI/quicktips

- Making your website accessible for people with a learning disability: www.intrasolutions.co.uk/website accessibility.pdf

- Using Widgit to make sites accessible: www.widgit.com/online/index.htm

## Reflection

1 Take a look at an accessible website and one that has not been made accessible. See 'Further reading and resources' for a list of websites.

2 Imagine you are writing a review for a magazine.

- What do you like or dislike about the websites?

- How have they been made accessible and how could they be made more accessible?

Speechmark

# Part 2
# Including and involving me

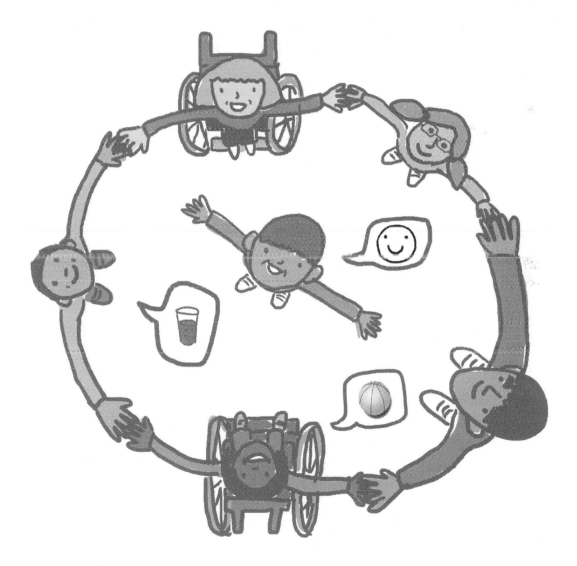

This part provides a set of tools that enable communication partners and services to support people with a learning disability to actively participate and be involved in their lives.

# Developing communication opportunities for people with complex needs

This section is about how we understand and support communication with people who are considered hard to reach. This may include people who are described as having profound and multiple learning disabilities (PMLD), severe learning disabilities or complex needs.

People with complex needs may have limited intentional communication skills, or may not yet be able to communicate intentionally and rely on others to interpret pre-intentional responses to internal or external stimuli which are associated with well-being.

Pre-intentional responses may be communicated through involuntary gestures, facial expressions, movements, sounds, changes in breathing or pulse rate, eye contact or laughter. Responses may also be voluntary such as refusing more food, reaching for something that is wanted or showing affection. Responses are considered pre-intentional until the person understands that these actions influence the behaviour of other people.

Intentional communication occurs when a person has an idea that they want to express, decides how they would like to express it, and then tries to do so. Intentional communication requires patterns of learned behaviour where a link between cause and effect is understood and an action is taken in order to gain a desired reaction. This may be achieved through conscious gestures, facial expressions or sounds and behaviours, through to more complex methods such as signing, using objects of reference, pictures and maybe some words.

Other factors which can affect communication for this group of people may include physical or sensory impairments or other health issues. The degree of pain that someone is experiencing can also affect a person's desire to communicate. These factors need be considered when communicating with people as they may affect which communication tools are suitable. For example, signing may be difficult for someone with a physical impairment such as cerebral palsy; and someone who is visually impaired may benefit more from tactile communication resources such as objects of reference or tactile symbols rather than pictures or visual symbols.

## Establishing and recording existing communication

The starting point for communicating with people with complex needs is to gain an understanding of how they already communicate and to use these methods to communicate with them.

Observation is the most important tool in establishing and recording communication. This can be achieved in the following ways.

- Simply spending time with the person.

- Interacting meaningfully with the person during care routines (routines such as bathing, washing and personal care should not be rushed as they provide ideal opportunities for communication and increasing the person's control).

- Observing how the person reacts in different circumstances, in different places and with different people.

- Engaging in activities.

- Engaging in play.

- Looking for subtle differences and nuances of expression.

- Observing physiological responses such as depth and rate of breathing, levels of energy, movement, posture, skin tone.

- Building a picture of what something might mean to a person, what is important and what they enjoy, through their responses.

An accurate picture of a person's communication methods can be built by sharing observations and interpretations with other people who also know the person well and checking these against subsequent observations over a period of time. Communication methods can be recorded using a range of methods including descriptions, videos, multimedia profiles and photographs (see the section on documenting communication).

## Creating opportunities to communicate

Much of the time spent with people with complex needs focuses on the care they require, for example moving and handling, feeding, dressing, bathing and toileting. The time allocated for support may also be determined by these care support needs.

Other factors that affect how much practitioners communicate with someone may include how a job description is phrased or interpreted; practitioners communicating with each other (task-related or otherwise) rather than with the person; or through a lack of understanding or skills in communicating with people with complex needs.

© Martin Goodwin, Jennie Miller and Cath Edwards  Speechmark

## Reflection

1 Consider how you like people to communicate with you and involve you now.

2 If you lost your ability to communicate, and had difficulty doing things for yourself, how would you want people to engage with you?

Be imaginative in how you communicate and involve people. From the most mundane of activities, make opportunities that give the person a chance to have fun, enjoy the interaction and share control of activities. Try not to feel self-conscious or worry about activities being age-appropriate because it is important to meet developmental needs and respond to a person's interests and the way they communicate.

Below are some ideas for creating opportunities to communicate.

- Engaging through play (regardless of age).

- Using sensory stimuli such as water, texture, sound, movement and light to gain response and interaction.

- Using art (especially sensory activities such as clay or plasticine modelling, hand and feet printing and collages).

- Supporting people in activities that stimulate the senses such as sensory rooms, swimming, being in the garden, visiting a farm, the countryside or the seaside.

- Sensory environments such as a room full of interactive technology or a sensory den made from homemade fabrics and other items and garden canes.

- Creating opportunities to express pleasure, preference, choice and requests.

- Creating opportunities to experience cause and effect ('If I do this, then this happens').

- Using objects of reference to support someone to know what is happening, to make choices and make requests (see the section on objects of reference).

- Using simple technological communication aids such as BIGmack™ to create cause and effect (see the section on using technology).

- Using music and rhythm (see the section on interactive approaches).

- Using dance, drama and movement (see the section on interactive approaches).

- Spending time using Intensive Interaction and other interactive approaches to communicate (see the section on interactive approaches).

Below are some factors that should be considered when communicating with people with complex needs.

- Value all communication and recognise that clear messages can also be communicated through non-verbal means.

- Pre-intentional behaviours should be responded to and given meaning.

- Behaviour, including behaviours that are challenging, can be a means of communication.

- Use methods that are appropriate to the person's ability.

- Methods may be adapted or tailored to meet individual needs.

- Use the communication methods that the person uses.

- Try different approaches, even if they have been tried before without apparent success.

- Consider the environment that you are in. Is there already too much sensory information? Is the environment noisy or busy? Is the television on? Are there a lot of distractions or people nearby? Is the person comfortable?

- Liaise with family and other people involved to gain a better understanding of communication. Share knowledge to support other people to communicate with the person.

- Give people time to respond by making sure that you pause between communication to enable the person to express a response or have a say in their own way.

Speechmark

## Reflection

1 Consider the activities that you currently engage in with a person who has complex needs. How could you promote better interaction and communication?

2 What activities could you introduce to create new opportunities for interaction and communication?

## Examples of good practice

A staff team supporting adults with complex needs in a short break setting recognised that much of their time was spent supporting people with their care needs. When this was discussed in a team meeting, they identified the ways in which positive communication and interaction was already promoted within routines and how this could be developed further. They also shared and listed activities that they had carried out and considered others that could be tried. It was agreed that support staff would ensure that opportunities to interact, engage and communicate would be recorded in the daily notes so that this time would be prioritised alongside care routines. At the next meeting, the team agreed that recording information around opportunities to interact, engage and communicate helped them to focus on this. Some staff members commented that they experienced greater job satisfaction as a result of the changes made.

Maggie is tube fed. Her support staff noticed that she was engaging in self-stimulating behaviour for long periods of time and it was difficult to meaningfully engage with her because there was little response. Her support staff realised that they could maximise the communication opportunities during this time by creating a sensory umbrella for her; she had a series of these for different times of the day. In the evening, she sat under a purple umbrella that was decorated with stars and moons that twinkled under the lights. Maggie responded to this by visually tracking movements. Support staff could use this stimulus to engage more meaningfully with her by using the umbrellas as part of her routine to interact with her and the represented objects.

A college supporting adults with complex needs uses multisensory stories to engage and involve students. Each sentence of the story is accompanied by a sensory action or object which is offered, and shared in turn while others are looking at other objects, to each member of a group. This enables people to experience and become involved in the story, promotes concentration, turn-taking and interaction with the storyteller and others who are involved in the story. Using sensory stimuli in storytelling also reinforces the meaning of written and spoken language. (See the video clip at www.pamis.org.uk/_page. php?id=24)

Paula would quite often be sleepy throughout the day because of the amount of medication that she was receiving. She would drift in and out of her sleep every few moments, making it difficult to engage her in any activity or to maintain communication for any period of time. Paula's support staff found this really difficult. During activities, while she was asleep, her support worker continued to stroke her hand and was ready to respond to continue the activity little by little whenever she woke up.

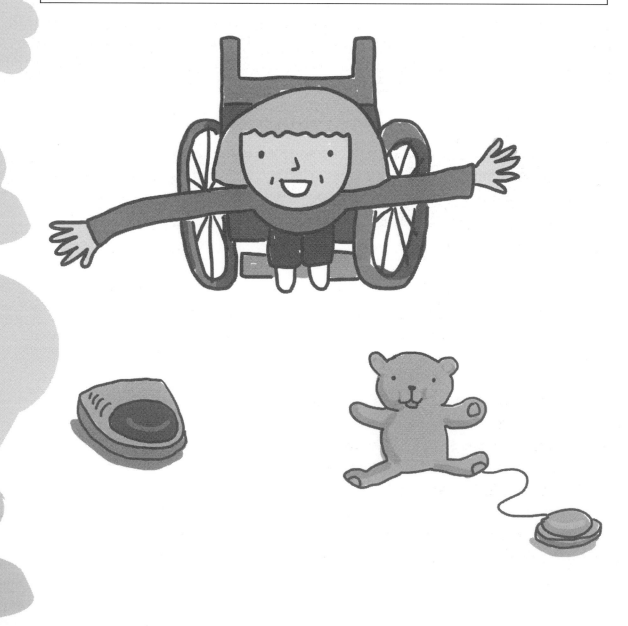

# Using pictures and symbols

Using pictures and symbols can enhance the opportunities to communicate with people, provided they have achieved this level of symbol development (see the section 'Enabling effective communication'). Using pictures and symbols can support people to communicate with others, access information, record information, be creative, make choices, follow instructions, anticipate what is about to happen, understand processes and routines, and become more involved. Using pictures and symbols can also support the development of social skills as people learn to approach and interact with other people and, as a result, interactions have more meaning.

It is important to consider that recognising symbols is a learning process like learning a new language. When preparing to create resources, the level of symbolic development that a person has should be considered so that the appropriate images are used. A person may be familiar with symbols that they use frequently but unable to recognise symbols for other, even related concepts, or more abstract symbols. It is therefore common that resources use a mixture of images across the symbolic development range. Resources designed for groups may use more than one image for more complex concepts: for example, photographs in addition to symbols. The use of images in resources may also be designed to support symbolic development from simpler images to more complex and abstract ones.

Photographs can easily be used as a communication resource using digital cameras and quick printing techniques. Photographs provide a great way of capturing the closest thing to an object in a more versatile format. When using photographs, it is important that the images best capture or represent what we want to communicate.

Photographs should be clear and taken from an aspect that is familiar to the person. The size, brightness and clarity of the focus should also be considered when using photographs. Photographs can be supported by symbols or words to aid association.

Symbols are visual representations of a word or concept. They should be clear and simple, representing small, unambiguous pieces of information which can be built up to form more complex pieces of information with more meaning. Symbols can range from being very pictorial, and most closely representing the original, to those that are more simplified and stylised. For example, a picture of a chair could be represented showing all four legs and appear to have depth and perspective or with only two legs, which is much more abstract. For more information on using photos and symbols at the appropriate symbolic level of development, please refer to the section 'Enabling effective communication'.

Consider how symbols are represented when making information accessible. Adding symbols to a document does not automatically make it more accessible if the individual has not yet attained the level of symbolic development required to recognise concepts in such an abstract form. It may be more appropriate to use photographs instead.

Also remember that people have to be taught how to understand symbols, especially those used to convey grammatical concepts such as 'before', 'in', 'on' or 'who', which rely on schematical concepts and rules that are more abstract. Verbs (action words) enable people to expand and explain more clearly and should be taught alongside descriptive words.

## Types of symbols

The most commonly used symbol communication systems are Makaton, Widgit Literacy Symbols, Picture Communication Symbols® (PCS), Change Picture Bank, Inspired Clip Art and Photos, and Photosymbols. These are described below.

- Widgit Literacy Symbols and software are designed specifically to support written information in print, on-screen and online as well as developing literacy and communication. Following the same structure as written language, users can learn to read and write with Widgit in much the same way as with words, as each word is represented by a symbol. Text can literally be translated into Widgit symbols (or other permissible symbols or photos that individuals can integrate into the software). Care must be taken to ensure that any differences in word meaning are correctly translated and that sentences have a simple structure. Widgit produces a range of software to support practitioners to make communication accessible and to support individuals with their literacy.

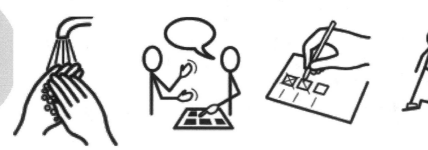

*Examples of Widgit Literacy Symbols (available in colour) for 'wash hands', 'communicate', 'fill in form' and 'goal' (Source: Widgit Symbols © Widget Software 2002–2015. www.widgit.com)*

- Makaton symbols were first published in 1985 and are used to provide visual support for objects and the written word. Makaton symbols continue to be developed in line with Makaton signs, as a core vocabulary graded into developmental stages. Makaton also provides additional topic vocabulary to support everyday activities. Makaton has a complementary bank of symbols which are simple and pictographic.

- Picture Communication Symbols® (PCS) was developed by Mayer-Johnson to be used with both high- and low-tech communication systems. These symbols tend to be more pictographic and detailed and there is less reliance on the need to learn the meanings of more abstract symbols. PCS offers a core library of around 5,000 symbols which can then be supplemented by more specialist symbols that are subject or language specific.

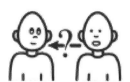 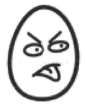 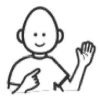 

*Examples of PCS symbols (available in colour) for 'ask', 'don't like', 'I want' and 'understand' (Source: The Picture Communication Symbols © 1981–2015 by Mayer-Johnson LLC, a Tobii Dynavox company. All Rights Reserved Worldwide. Used with permission. Boardmaker® is a trademark of Mayer-Johnson LLC)*

- Change Picture Bank was developed by Change, an organisation run by people with learning disabilities. The Change Picture Bank is an extensive set of images that describe a range of situations and contexts in areas such as health, criminal justice, independent living, employment and other areas of life. Change Picture Bank images can easily be put into documents.

- Photosymbols was developed by Photosymbols Ltd. It provides an extensive range of photographs which are produced using staged photography that is clear and simple and represents situations and concepts. Examples include a photograph for getting up, taking blood pressure, having a scan, choosing clothes, having a chat and bowling. Photosymbols help people to understand situations and contexts in a wide range of daily living activities. Photosymbols can easily be put into documents.

- Inspired Easy Read Clip Art and Inspired Easy Read Photo collection have been developed by Inspired Services Publishing. The Inspired Easy Read Clip Art Collection uses an extensive range of clear colour drawings that describe a range of situations and contexts in areas of life such as access, buildings, places, education, children and families, and health. The Inspired Easy Read Photo Collection uses an extensive range of photographs that capture specific situations and contexts such as using an ATM or visiting the library.

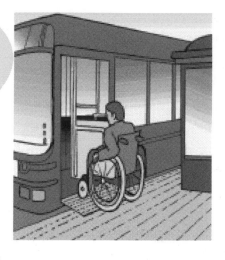
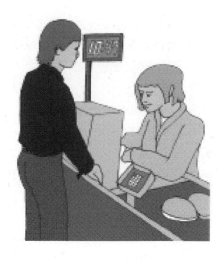

*Examples of Inspired Easy Read Clip Art (available in colour) for 'accessible bus'
and 'supermarket checkout' (Source: Inspired Easy Read Clip Art Collection © Inspired Pics.
Available from: www.inspired.pics)*

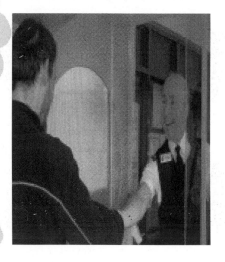
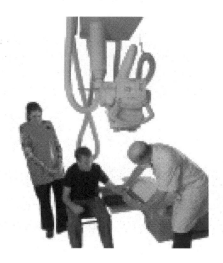

*Examples of Inspired Easy Read Photos (available in colour) for 'police station enquiry' and 'X-ray arm'
(Source: Inspired Easy Read Clip Art Collection © Inspired Pics. Available from: www.inspired.pics)*

Some other systems are Symbolstix, which is an online resource of stick figures and symbols originally designed for an internet weekly newspaper *News-2-You*; Snaps, by Smartbox Assistive Technology, which is a photo library; and See Sense, which is a small picture library.

All of the above symbol systems can be either purchased or downloaded free of charge from the internet (see the website references in 'Further reading and resources').

## Reflection

1 Draw your own symbols for the following words:
- happy
- me
- hospital
- dog
- why
- old
- hungry.

2  See whether other people can understand your symbols.

Consider what worked well or didn't work.

## Using symbols and pictures in the environment

Picture and symbol immersion is a method of supporting people to make associations between pictures or symbols and what they represent. It involves simply displaying pictures or symbols of objects, activities, rooms or areas appropriately around an environment, such as a college, day service or nursery. The same symbols are used when referring to those objects, areas or activities; for making choices; requesting to use items; and when engaging in activities or going to specific places. People are supported to make associations through repetition and use. For example, a picture or symbol for a toilet is shown (maybe in a key-ring) before a person is supported to go to the toilet and then shown again on the toilet door.

Matching activities can also be used to reinforce associations. For example, matching a picture or symbol cards with items on a table; treasure hunt games using a picture or symbol (which is brought back); or two pictures or symbols to represent what can be found (eg a sweet) in an area or a room (on the table or in the kitchen).

## Using pictures and symbols as a personal communication aid

Communication books are a method of enabling a person to have access to the pictures and symbols that they use, so that they can freely communicate with others. The person is able to point to or select pictures or symbols to make requests, express feelings, thoughts, ideas, and so on. These books should be personalised according to the person's ability and interests.

PECS (Picture Exchange Communication System) is a more structured communication approach to support people to initiate and develop communication. It was originally developed for use with children but is effective for people of all ages. It is not expensive to implement or use but it does require training and resources. People are initially taught to exchange a picture for something that they want, for example a drink; they then move on to choose between pictures, which supports choice. Following this, people learn how to use pictures to construct sentences to make requests such as 'I want the book' or make a comment such as 'I can see the car'. Language is then expanded to include more complex structures such as adjectives: 'I want the red book'; verbs: 'the girl is running'; and prepositions: 'the book is on the table'. The approach also supports people to express how they feel or what their opinion is about something.

## Using pictures and symbols to make information easier to understand

When using pictures and/or symbols to make information accessible, consider the following factors.

- Whether the information is for one individual or several people and what their level of symbolic development is.

- Whether a mixture of photos or symbols helps the person or just one type.

- The layout used: does it help the person more if the symbols or pictures are at the side, on top or underneath words?

- The amount of information there is on one page.

- The language used: are the concepts easy to understand?

- How it flows and whether this is in a logical and sequential order.

- The number of items that are used; can the person process information easily?

- Whether the person understands the pictures or symbols that are used.

- Do the pictures or symbols used best represent the message?

- Are photos clear?

© Martin Goodwin, Jennie Miller and Cath Edwards · Speechmark

## Reflection

Consider how you already use pictures and symbols:

- How are they used to support people to communicate with you?

- How are they used to support you to communicate with other people?

- How effective is the use of pictures and symbols?

## Examples of good practice

A support service produces flyers to promote upcoming events and activities. These are made accessible using pictures and symbols that represent the activity and event alongside words.

Symbol immersion is used in a play setting to tell children which play opportunities are taking place in various rooms. The same symbols are used on choice boards, symbol key-rings and the timetable. Children are also supported to use these to make choices or requests.

Symbols are used within a residential home to label activities of daily living and key aspects of routine. In appropriate areas of the bathroom there are symbols for having a bath or shower, washing hair, brushing teeth and using the toilet. In the bedroom, there are symbols on the wardrobe for getting dressed and drying hair at the dresser. The same symbols are used on a key-ring to talk about what is going to happen next in the routine. Practitioners at the residential home felt that this made people feel much more involved in their personal routines and enabled people to anticipate what was happening next. They found that the people they supported engaged more in the process, which became less of a routine that was done 'to' or 'for' them and more of a routine that was done 'with' them.

Sarah's support worker has taken a series of photographs of different places and activities that are part of Sarah's routine or that she enjoys doing. These are used when supporting Sarah to understand where she is going (eg day service, the doctor's, shopping) or to support her to make choices about where she wants to go and what she would like to do (café, cinema, walking, cycling, picnic in the park).

# Person-centred planning approaches

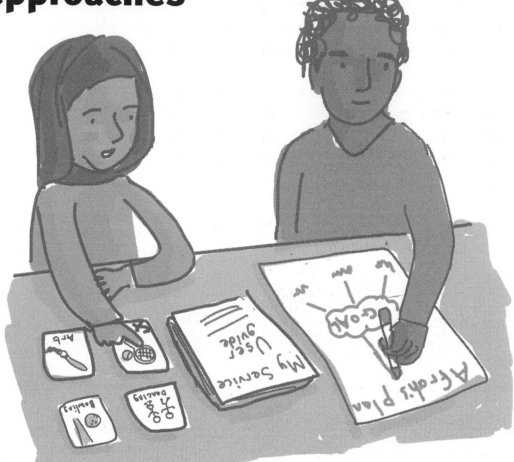

> "Person-centred planning is a way of helping people who want to make some changes in their life. It is an empowering approach to helping people plan their future and organise the support and services they need. It seeks to mirror the ways in which 'ordinary people' make plans."

(Sanderson et al, 1997, p13)

Traditionally, processes involving assessment are service-orientated, conducted by services and professionals and focus on aims and goals that are considered to be important to them. When this is the case, the control and power in these processes is held by services, not by the individual being supported. Person-centred approaches aim to shift the balance of this power by putting the individual at the centre of this process and enabling them, if wished, to establish their own personalised support and use of a range of settings and community networks.

Person-centred planning is based on values of the social model of disability and inclusion. Instead of fitting people into services, person-centred planning starts with the person and asks what is important to them and how they want to live their life; it then works on finding ways to make this possible. Apart from the individual, other people who are involved in the planning process may include parents, siblings, friends and advocates as well as (but not always) people who are paid to support them.

Person-centred planning consists of a range of creative approaches that enable people to introduce themselves to others, discover and communicate what is important to them, consider what their support needs are and what they want in their present and future. The approaches support people to think about short and longer term goals and plan how to achieve these.

Person-centred thinking means ensuring that support is based on what is important to the person. It is about sharing power with the person and committing to changing situations they are not happy with. Person-centred thinking can mean a significant shift in value base and a re-evaluation of how assessments are made and how services are delivered.

The most commonly used person-centred planning approaches are:

- PATH, developed by Jack Pearpoint, Marsha Frost and John O'Brien

- Maps, developed by Judith Snow, Jack Pearpoint, Marsha Frost and John O'Brien

- Essential Lifestyle Planning, developed by Michael Smull and Susan Burke-Harrison

- Personal Futures Planning, developed by Beth Mount and John O'Brien

- Individual Service Design, developed by Jack Yates and his colleagues.

For a comprehensive guide to the background and use of these approaches, along with practical guidance and examples, see Helen Sanderson and Associates' book *People, Plans and Possibilities* (1997). It was written in response to what was learned from research in the UK with people who have learning disability around their experiences of planning and how they would like things to be done differently. These planning styles use creative techniques such as graphic facilitation, pictures, symbols and photographs to make them accessible and can be recorded in a variety of formats such as DVDs, scrapbooks and posters. Person-centred plans belong to and are kept by the person; copies may also be kept by those who support them.

## Reflection

1 Think about your morning routine. Which aspects of it are essential, which are important, and which are more of a matter of personal preference? (For example, it is essential to snooze for 10 minutes before getting out of bed; it is important to have a cup of tea, but not the end of the world if you have coffee; it would be your preference to wake up next to ...).

2 Consider someone you support. What do you think she or he would say was essential, important, or their preference?

3 If you were being supported in your morning routine, what would you want people to know?

4 How might someone with a learning disability tell you how they like to be supported in the morning?

## Example of good practice

Nona lives in a supported tenancy. Her behaviour was challenging to the people who supported her and her family were becoming increasingly concerned that these behaviours were isolating her from activities and experiences that she used to enjoy.

Nona's key worker had recently done some training in person-centred planning approaches and decided to support Nona to write an Essential Lifestyle Plan. The people who contributed to Nona's plan included Nona herself, her brother (who also has a learning disability), her mother, two members of staff from the day service and staff from home. The first stage involved supporting Nona to visit these people and talk about what they liked about Nona and what she was good at. Nona enjoyed this and she began to show more interest in her plan. Nona's key worker realised that, over recent months, when people talked to Nona about herself, the focus had been on her behaviours and had been quite negative. Talking about positive things helped everybody focus on Nona and who she was. Nona was supported to make a poster and used photographs and pictures to illustrate the quotes of what people had said about her. Every time someone came into her room, she asked them to read something from the poster!

Speechmark

The next stage involved working with Nona to think about what was important to her, what she enjoyed doing and how she liked to be supported. The plan showed that staff were not supporting Nona consistently and support was very task-focused because of people's caution due to her aggression towards them. It showed that it was really important to Nona that staff knocked on her door and waited to be invited in before entering; that she liked to have a bath in the evening instead of the morning, so she could spend more time having her hair done and nails painted instead of rushing to dress and get out (which made her angry); that it was important to her to be able to change her clothes several times during the day; that the activities that she was involved in at the day centre were not what she enjoyed; and that she wanted to spend more time going out with Mum. The way in which her support staff at home supported Nona changed as they were engaged in talking about positive things.

Positive relationships developed as support staff spent more time with her doing activities such as nail painting, which Nona enjoyed. Changes were made at the day service and Mum took her out on alternate Saturday afternoons. Nona became much more settled and was less aggressive towards staff as their relationships improved.

# Exploring social situations through stories

Stories are a method that has been used for generations to support people to gain a greater understanding of their environment, experiences and social situations.

We use stories in everyday life; this adds to our understanding of other people's experiences and influences how we might behave in similar situations. Examples include:

- recalling experiences and events from our own lives for our friends and family

- anecdotes in our conversations to help other people understand what we are saying

- reading factual stories in newspapers or magazines

- watching the news or documentaries

- reading fictional stories

- watching films or soap operas.

Exploring social situations through stories has been developed as a method of supporting children and adults with a learning disability to better understand and process social situations and to understand social rules, conventions and dynamics that they may find difficult to understand. Carol Gray has written extensive guidance on writing Social Stories™ and we recommend that you read her useful guidance on how to put a social story together (see www.thegraycenter.org). Stories are especially useful when supporting people who find information easier to understand if it is presented in a concrete and structured way that is applicable to their life.

Nicola Grove and OpenStoryTellers (www.openstorytellers.org.uk) have developed an approach called 'Storysharing®' (detailed in Grove, 2014; Grove, 2012). The approach is also explained under the title 'Personal Narratives' in Grove, 2009. Storysharing is a way of supporting people with learning disabilities to tell stories about things that have happened in their lives, both 'significant events and/or everyday happenings' (Grove, 2009, p27) by 'developing the recall and sharing of personal experiences' (Mencap, 2011, p54).

The approach relies on communication partners supporting the person to recall and tell to one person or a small group an anecdote about their life. Anecdotes could include 'the day I made a cake and I dropped it', 'the time I went to hospital', 'going to the football match' or 'putting hair gel on to go to the party'. Storysharing enables the person's experience to be relived and re-encountered by sharing it with others. This involves an appropriate level of support from the communication partner, ranging from simply helping the person to rehearse the story verbally, to use of technology such as a BIGmack™, key objects, photos or other communication devices, to co-active telling.

Sharing the story with others can help a person to 'recall and understand experience' (Grove, 2014, p7), to gain a fuller sense of identity and to have a voice in their own lives. A wider circle of people can also learn what matters to the person and how they like to live their life. This can importantly help the communication partner to listen to and further involve the person in making choices and decisions about their life.

Stories may be used to develop an understanding of actions. For example:

- with a child in a play setting where they find it difficult to share and then fail to understand why they may not be popular with other children

- to support people to understand a process such as moving house or going to a new school

- to support people to understand changes such as those that are or will be happening to an adolescent body

- to support people to make sense of difficult subjects, for instance news items such as natural disasters and war

- to support people to understand experiences before an event, such as a party or an operation, or experiences after an event, such as injury or good experiences on holiday.

Stories can be presented like a story book. The story has a practical objective which is to support the person to gain a better understanding of social situations so that, over time, a person's behaviour may change or their anxiety may reduce in situations or experiences that distress them, or their behaviour is reinforced where experiences have been positive.

It is possible to purchase stories around common or major issues; stories can also be constructed specifically for individuals and around their situation or issue, and tailored to meet the communication needs of the individual, using photographs or references to familiar people, places and objects. When writing a story, consider the following factors.

- Sentences should be constructed carefully and objectively to support the person to process information. Stories should have a clear, concise and accurate structure about what is happening in one social situation.

- Use positive language and incorporate what the person already does well. Reinforce that it is all right for certain things to happen or for people to react in a certain way, if this is so.

- Stories should make the person feel comfortable and good about what they do well, as well as working on the issue that needs support.

- Stories describe what may seem obvious to most of us, but can aid the understanding of a situation by someone with learning disability.

- The story should describe the situation and/or environment, what happens and why, and how people respond and why; it may suggest appropriate responses for the person to make.

- Stories should be motivating and appropriate to the level of understanding of the person. Cartoon strips and articles, for example, are a good way of making stories more age-appropriate to teenagers and adults but they can be more difficult to follow.

- The information should not be overwhelming to the person by including information that is not relevant to the situation. The story may only contain one point per page.

- Stories can be written in the first person to help the person imagine themselves in the situation. Stories can be personalised further by using the person's name or pictures of the person (where this would be positive, eg 'Sam's holiday').

- The story should be made accessible by using communication methods that the person already uses, for example pictures and symbols.

- Consider when the story should be read, how often and with whom.

Be creative about the media that you use; stories don't have to be in book form. The following formats may also be considered.

- Cartoon strips may be more acceptable to teenagers or young people than story books.

- Magazine style articles may be more engaging to some people.

- Interviews about people's experiences – a group might be supported to interview people about how they felt when they experienced something, eg moving house, leaving school, losing or breaking something of value.

- Drama – taking turns to take different roles in a social situation (eg bullying) and then talking about how it felt. Consider using props, objects of reference or BIGmack™ to support a person to tell their own narrative.

- A story board showing pictures or photographs demonstrating a sequence of events.

- Conversation – chatting about experiences and responses informally or following a set pattern (see the example below).

- Arts and crafts – through other artists' work and by supporting people to express their own experiences through art.

- Poetry – again through other people's work and by supporting people to express their own experiences through poetry.

- Story bag or sensory story – a collection of objects with guidance that helps the communication partner to use the objects to put together a story that conveys the issue.

- Film, soap opera and theatre – where people's life experiences and responses are enacted.

## Reflection

1 Consider social situations that people whom you work with find difficult.

2 Consider how you could use stories to explore these social situations.

## Examples of good practice

John attends an after-school play group. He found it very difficult to share and would hit other children when he was told to share toys or when another child wanted a toy from him. To help John understand, his play leader created a story that made him aware of the importance of sharing toys with friends and how other children felt if he did not share.

Amir becomes very anxious when situations are not familiar to him and he doesn't know what to expect. When his Dad died, Amir's community support worker, who knew him and his family well, used storytelling methods to support Amir through the process of the funeral, why people were behaving differently and why certain routines had changed in his life.

Valerie finds it very difficult to understand that there is more than one way of doing something and that it is acceptable for other people do things in a different way from the way that she chooses. Moving into a shared house with a team of support staff highlighted endless differences between the way Valerie carried out tasks and the way other people achieved the same thing. The anxiety that this caused Valerie was constant and was beginning to cause violent and aggressive outbursts towards her co-tenant and support staff.

Following a meeting, the staff team agreed on an approach to reinforce that it is okay for Valerie to do something her way and it is equally acceptable for other people to do the same thing in a different way. The approach involved all team members following the same pattern, or story. In conversation, support staff would point out something that someone else was doing in everyday situations on the television, on the bus, while shopping, etc and observe that this differed from how they did it, but this was okay too because different people do things in different ways sometimes. While Valerie was relaxed, they would also talk to her about something that she was doing, reinforce that it was a good way of doing it and maybe comment that they had seen someone else doing the same thing in a completely different way, but this was also a good way of doing it for them.

Over time, Valerie became less anxious about how other people carried out everyday tasks at home and her aggressive outbursts stopped. When she did become anxious, a reminder following the pattern set by the support staff would be enough to reduce her anxiety.

Emma is going on holiday next month. To help prepare her for the inevitable changes in her routine and the new experiences she will encounter, her family have put together a series of story boards. Each story board addresses a different situation, such as 'packing', 'the airport', 'flying', and 'in the hotel', so that Emma becomes familiar with what is going to happen and what she can expect. 'At the airport', for example, includes situations such as queuing, showing passports, allowing her bag to be scanned, being able to look around the shops and waiting patiently. Her family take the story boards with them.

Susanna communicates mainly with her eyes; she has very limited movement of limbs and face and it is difficult for her to engage beyond one-to-one interactions. As part of a Storysharing group, Susanna joined in with telling stories about things that happen in her family. It was so motivating for her to share the tale of being woken up by her father's snores that she began to independently move her hand to operate a BIGmack™ communication aid (onto which another group member had recorded a loud snore!). Her family were thrilled with her progress.

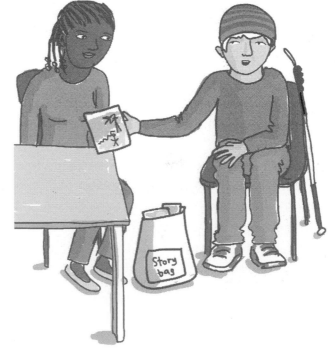

© Martin Goodwin, Jennie Miller and Cath Edwards

# Graphic facilitation

Graphic facilitation is a process of graphically representing words, ideas and concepts through drawn images. This approach may be used before supporting a person (eg in documents or stories); during support (eg in meetings or when planning with someone); or after an event (eg making the minutes of meetings accessible).

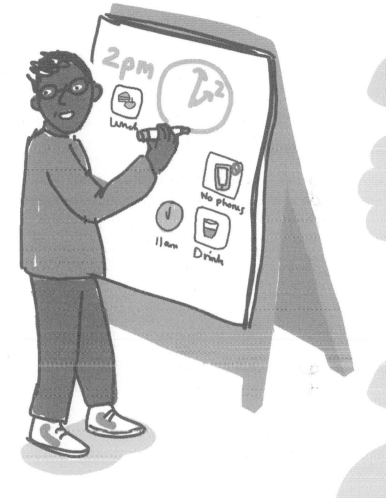

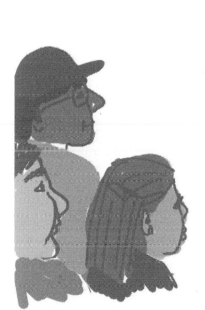

Graphic facilitation may use drawings mixed with symbols to represent key concepts. There are conventions that can be learned to make images clearer, such as the use of arrows to connect ideas or demonstrate flow and sequence, dream clouds representing wishes and speech bubbles representing what people say. There are also images that can be learned such as representations of people, places and key concepts that simplify both the facilitation and understanding of graphics. Training in graphic facilitation is advisable (either formally or self-directed).

The advantages of using graphic facilitation include:

- making information easier to understand
- encouraging people to be involved in their meetings
- keeping people focused on what is being discussed
- helping people to remember what has been discussed earlier in the meeting
- it is a permanent and accessible record of what has been discussed or agreed
- it enables feelings as well as ideas to be recorded
- it shows a connection between ideas
- it's fun!

When using graphic facilitation, it is important that:

- Preparation is done in advance for key graphics that are likely to be needed (such as the structure or titles) while allowing for the process to be jointly carried out.

- If colours are used, these aid understanding, for example by showing different ideas or themes.

- Graphics are clear and easy to understand, are appropriate in the context and not ambiguous or abstract.

- Graphics are used appropriately alongside text.

- The facilitator takes into consideration the stage of symbolic development of the person or people for whom it is intended.

- Graphic facilitation should add meaning and support understanding and involvement.

- A shared meaning and interpretation takes place by discussing and involving people in the design or use of pictures to represent concepts or issues.

Graphic facilitation can be more difficult for some people to understand because they may need a more consistent representation (such as a symbol or photograph). It may be confusing for some people to understand freely drawn images that may or may not look the same. Communication partners should consider the stage of symbolic development that a person or audience has achieved.

## Reflection

Plan an evening's entertainment for friends, using coloured pens to represent your ideas graphically on a big sheet of paper.

- How easy did you find this?

- What worked well and what did you struggle with?

## Examples of good practice

During her review, Barbara's social worker used graphic facilitation to record what was being discussed. He had prepared an agenda using graphic facilitation which used images, including a house for home issues, a building with people in it for day services and college, a green cross for health and coins for finances. He started the review by drawing a person in the middle of a large sheet of paper, coloured her clothes the same as Barbara's and wrote her name underneath. He then drew small people underneath this to represent the other people at the meeting and added their names. He drew an arrow to the first subject area and illustrated the discussion by using happy and sad faces for what Barbara said was working or not working, empty boxes for actions to do and ticked boxes for actions taken since the last review. Previously, Barbara had quickly become bored during reviews. However, using graphic facilitation in the review helped her to be more involved, contribute more and to concentrate on what was being said.

An after-school group for young people with learning disabilities uses graphic facilitation when planning a project or an event. All the ideas suggested are put in bubbles within an arrow that fills the sheet of paper. At the head of the arrow are images representing the project or event.

Letters and meeting minutes sent out by an advocacy group are written using simple language and graphics to help members understand its contents.

When consulting with a group of service users about how to improve the day service, the group was supported to record their ideas by a graphic facilitator who represented what was discussed throughout the meeting. The graphics were also used in the report produced at the end of the consultation process to show what was discussed and what actions were taken.

# Interactive approaches

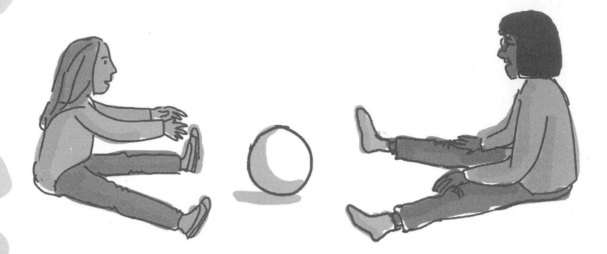

Interactive approaches are a process of making contact and building relationships with people who do not use words to communicate. These approaches have been developed for use with people who are still at the very early stages of communication development. Some of the techniques can also be useful with people who have acquired some speech but need to develop further skills in areas such as making eye contact and turn-taking. As well as a method of developing communication skills, interactive approaches are a way of enjoying being with and building a positive relationship with someone whose learning disabilities are more severe or complex.

Intensive Interaction is an approach introduced by the psychologist Geraint Ephraim and developed by Dave Hewett and Melanie Nind in the 1980s at Harperbury Hospital School in Hertfordshire, UK. They realised that, for some people, learning to be with someone and interacting socially was more important than the traditional approach to teaching people with learning disabilities, which focused on behavioural techniques and promoting independence skills. By the 1990s, Intensive Interaction gained wider recognition across the UK with one of its leading advocates, Phoebe Caldwell, who had also worked alongside Geraint Ephraim, helping to promote the approach.

Intensive Interaction is a particularly valuable process. People whose learning disabilities are profound or complex can be socially isolated, existing in a world of their own, stimulating themselves through movement, such as hand flapping and rocking; vocalisations and other sounds made, for example, by tapping or banging; and through touching themselves or their environment.

Speechmark

The process of Intensive Interaction begins with observing a person and the rituals that have meaning to them. The communication partner (the person supporting the individual) makes themselves interesting by engaging in (non-harmful) activities that the individual understands and already carries out. Once the communication partner has the person's attention, they vary the response they make to engage the person.

This may be achieved by:

- altering the sound by elongating it, changing the note or intonation, adding another small sound or movement

- changing the movement slightly by altering the rhythm, direction or size of the movement, adding sound

- tapping out a similar or different rhythm, tapping on a different surface, adding another sound or movement.

Over time, the opportunities created by the practitioner become a form of mutual communication and the turn-taking between two people becomes a conversation that both are engaged in. Solitary stimulation: 'I do something and it feels like this' gradually becomes a shared activity: 'I do something and they enjoy doing this too'. These positive interactions are a way of enjoying spending time together and building up a relationship.

Through Intensive Interaction the person may learn to:

- Understand cause and effect

- Anticipate and seek responses

- Take turns

- Imitate

- Gain and hold attention

- Initiate eye contact and touch

- Show interest in others

- Enjoy interaction.

(*Source*: Nind & Hewett, 2005)

Over time, people may begin to anticipate responses and seek this by initiating communication through approaching the communication partner or responding to interactions in deeper and more meaningful ways.

Intensive Interaction is about understanding how a person communicates and interacting with them. The process demonstrates respect for who the person is and how they communicate. It involves spending a lot of time engaging with the person, during which the aim is for the person to respond to and actively enjoy the process of interaction and communication. The whole process is led by the person, with the communication partner observing what motivates them and gently exploring opportunities for interaction.

## Reflection

Search for 'intensive interaction video clip' on the internet.

- What do you see the worker doing?

- How do they join in with the person?

- How could you use this approach to engage with the people you support?

Intensive Interaction principles can be carried out through different activities or media to enable the development of communication, interaction and fun with people. These are sometimes termed interactive approaches and may include using art forms such as music, movement, drama, story and art.

Any stimulus has interactive possibilities, so be creative about how you use activities or media to engage with people. For example:

- take turns blowing bubbles

- copying and making different movements while jumping or running through puddles in the park

- exploring paint or salt dough physically with someone

- using kitchen items as percussion instruments – copying, slightly adapting sounds, creating rhythms with someone, turn-taking

- using finger puppets to explore the exchange of communication.

The key elements of interactive approaches are:

- turn-taking

- engaging in an activity alongside or directly with a person

- giving people time to respond, even if this feels awkward

- copying or reflecting back what someone is doing

- repeating opportunities to explore stimulus and interact through it

- developing an understanding of each other

- becoming aware of each other's presence

- allowing the person to shape the process themselves

- observing and noticing responses to stimuli

- hooking into a person's preferences, what they find interesting and motivating

- offering possibilities that extend or sustain a person's interest.

## Examples of good practice

When one of the authors started working with people with a learning disability and was introduced to the people they would be working with, two men were having a conversation which sounded something like this

First person: 'Ahoooooooooow, oh!'

Second person: 'Ahooooooooooooooooooooooooooooow, oh, oh!'

First person: 'Ahoooooooooow, oh!'

Second person: 'Ahooooooooooooooooooooooooooooow, oh, oh, oh!'

and so on, with increasing enthusiasm and volume on both parts. It wasn't until later that day that the author realised that one of the men was not a service user but a manager! In this environment, the sounds that people made were all part of their joint vocabulary. Conversations such as this occurred regularly and alongside any other activity and were initiated by both the individual and/or support staff.

Conrad is a child with autism; he does not communicate verbally. It had always been really difficult to gain Conrad's attention to engage with him. His support worker had been using Intensive Interaction techniques to relate to Conrad and gain his attention. Conrad enjoyed fast-forwarding and rewinding DVDs to watch and rewatch the same few scenes, which held his attention for minutes at a time. After spending some time watching some scenes from *Popeye*, Conrad's support worker made an impression of some of the voices of the characters for Conrad and found that this captured his attention and gained eye contact. Conrad's support worker then began to create a bank of sounds that Conrad found engaging, including different voices and songs with 'silly' sounds, which captured his attention. Over time, an increasing interactive rapport was developed with Conrad by having fun in exploring sounds.

Isobel can use a few words and is communicative with her facial expressions and posture. During a den-building activity, Isobel was offered fabrics to choose. Reaching for a gold net fabric, she lifted it as though trying to put it on her head. The adult helped her drape it over her head and then took her to a large wall mirror so that she could see the effect. Isobel kept making eye contact through the net, so the adult joined her underneath it and together they improvised and sustained a game of peep-bo.

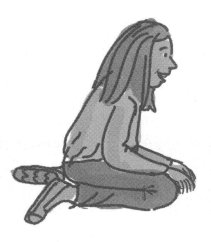
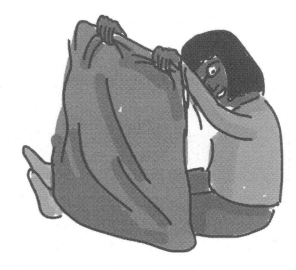

 Speechmark

# Choice boards

Choice boards allow a person to indicate choices or request items by pointing to a representation of their choice. How that choice is represented will depend on how that person communicates. Boards can be tailored to individual communication needs by using objects of reference, pictures, photographs, symbols or words (or a combination), depending on the individual's level of symbolic development. The visual nature of a choice board relies less on a person's memory and can support people to initiate choice.

Choice boards typically show a range of pictures or symbols on a grid. The number of options will depend on the ability of the individual and the number of choices available at that time. Some people find too many choices overwhelming initially, so additional choices may be added over time or stay at a two or three option level. It is important to consider whether the choices provided on the board are available. Some people may find it confusing or hard to accept that choices that are offered are then not available to them.

Choice can be indicated by, for example, pointing, eye gazing or nodding to an image that is pointed to. When introducing choices, it is best to start with a few options and then gradually increase them according to the person's ability. It is important to make sure that the person understands the item or event that is represented and that they like the objects or activities represented. Choice boards may also be more interactive, whereby the individual demonstrates their choice by moving an object of reference or a card from one area to another to demonstrate their choice. Objects of reference, printed pictures or symbols can be mounted using Velcro™ or Blu Tack™.

People can be supported to develop skills by gradually increasing the number of situations in which they are offered choices and by increasing the number of choices available.

Choice boards can be made easily and thereby tailored to individual communication needs. Boards may also be purchased. The GO TALK communication aids are available with different numbers of choice options depending on the ability of the individual. Increasingly, versions exist on tablet computers and smart phones which have the advantages of being portable and more readily available.

Think creatively about how you present choices. Formats such as fans or spinners could be used, for example. Fans have options on bookmark-sized cards fastened together using a paper fastener at one end. These cards can be displayed all together or one at a time as appropriate to support people to make choices. Spinners have choices, such as activities, displayed on segments of a circle. People can be supported to turn a pointer to the activity of their choice, or the pointer can be spun and the person can indicate whether they want to do that activity or not.

Talking Mats™ are another example of how people can be supported to make choices, particularly about a specific issue or topic. These were developed by Joan Murphy at the University of Stirling, UK. This communication tool uses a mat with symbols attached by Velcro. The mat is divided into sections that represent potential views, for example: happy, not sure, unhappy; working or not working; like, don't like. The person is then supported to put their choices in different categories. To be successful, a person needs to understand the significance of the different categories and what each symbol means. Talking mats can be used to support people to express preferences or views, plan for the future and in other areas such as service consultation.

## Reflection

Consider the choices that you regularly support people to make.

- Are there any situations where using a choice board to support this process would be beneficial?

- What options would you place on the choice board?

- How would this be presented to the person?

- How many choices would be appropriate for the person?

## Examples of good practice

At a day service, people are supported to choose the activity that they would like to take part in by using choice boards. A board is mounted on an easel with different activities shown (such as jigsaws, drawing, craft, using the computers, relaxing in the sensory room). There are objects of reference, photographs and symbols for each choice; the objects of reference are removable so that people can handle them.

The canteen at a college for students with learning disabilities offers menu choices on a board. People can indicate their choice of meal, drinks or snacks by pointing to the pictures.

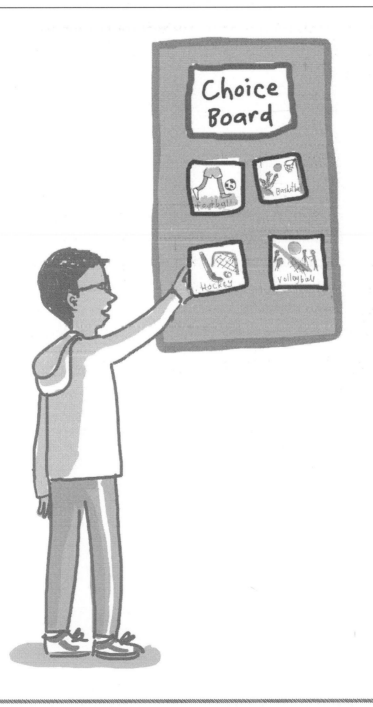

# Enabling choice and decision making

> **Offering opportunities to make choices 'is the start of a continuum that leads ultimately to being able to initiate communication, though [some people] may never achieve this level; it is also an important part of treating people in a respectful and inclusive way.**

(Goodwin & Edwards, 2009, p11)

It is well documented that people with a learning disability do not always share the same opportunities to make choices as the rest of society and it is often assumed that people who have no or little verbal communication cannot make choices or decisions.

Being able to make choices and act on them is something that most people take for granted: what time to get up in the morning, whether to get dressed before or after having breakfast, what to have for breakfast, what to wear, and so on, before considering more significant decisions such as where to live and with whom, which college to go to, or which government party to vote for. Most services and practitioners supporting people with a learning disability are involved in making decisions with or on behalf of the people they support.

The Mental Capacity Act 2005, which came into force in 2007 in the UK, is regarded as best practice even though it only legally applies to supporting people aged 16 and over. The Act supports people's rights to make their own decisions and provides guidance for when other people can make decisions on their behalf. It has challenged practitioners to consider how they support people to make choices and decisions that affect the lives of people with a learning disability.

The first three key principles of the Act are:

1   A person must be assumed to have capacity unless it is established that they lack capacity.

2   A person is not to be treated as unable to make a decision unless all practicable steps to help him/her to do so have been taken without success.

3   A person is not to be treated as unable to make a decision merely because he [or she] makes an unwise decision (Section 1, Mental Capacity Act 2005).

A person's capacity to make choices is decision-specific and time-specific. This means that because someone may lack capacity to make a decision about one issue, it does not mean that they lack the capacity to make other decisions. If a person lacks capacity now, this does not mean that they will lack capacity in the future.

The Act says that a person is unable to make a decision if he or she cannot:

- Understand the information relevant to the decision

- Retain that information

- Use or weigh that information as part of the process of making a decision, or

- Communicate the decision.

The ways in which we support people to understand information, make a decision and communicate this decision is the key to enabling that person to be involved in making decisions that affect their lives. The Mental Capacity Act is enforceable around choices such as medical treatment, finances and where to live; however, the principles are applicable to all choices including what to wear, choosing from a menu, which sofa to buy and which sessions to attend at day service.

For some people with learning disabilities, making choices, even simple ones, can be a difficult process. This requires an ability to understand context, remember choice options, be able to consider more than one choice at a time, understand what choices represent and be able to intentionally communicate preference.

When supporting someone to make choices and decisions, it may be helpful to consider the following factors.

- There may be a need to understand the concept of time to make some choices and decisions. Daily choices are easier for some people to make because they are in the here and now (concrete) and the consequence of making that choice is immediate (for example, choosing which jumper to wear). Choices that do not relate to the immediate present and may not happen until the distant future (abstract) are more difficult to understand, such as which clothes to choose to wear on holiday or what to do next Saturday. When supporting people to make choices and decisions, it may also be necessary to support someone to understand time order and sequence.

- Remember that people with learning disabilities may have limited or negative experiences of being involved in making choices and decisions. It is important that people gain positive experience in making choices and that they have the opportunity to observe the cause-and-effect relationship between making a choice and the outcome.

- It is a normal part of learning to make choices that are wrong or unsuitable, or to change your mind once you realise the choice is not actually what you wanted.

- It is important that people develop confidence in making decisions; communication partners should respect and respond to people's choices, regardless of whether they agree with the choice or whether the outcome is 'successful' or 'right'. However, it is also important to support the person to not come to harm, especially when the person cannot predict the likely harm.

- Consider how you present choices. If this exceeds ability, it may be overwhelming. It is therefore important to understand a person's cognitive ability level, preferred methods of communication and experience.

- A person may be able to make a choice at one level for one thing but not at the same level for something else. For example, someone may be able to choose between having tea or coffee to drink when asked verbally, but may struggle to decide between lasagne and chicken for tea when this choice is also presented verbally. Difficulty in picturing these two options, which are less familiar to the person, means that it would be more appropriate for the second choice to be offered using less complex methods of communication such as pictures or the actual objects.

- Consider how a choice is presented. For example, someone may not be able to choose between having jam or marmalade on crumpets when they are asked out of context while doing a jigsaw puzzle in the living room; but the same choice presented within the activity of making the crumpets in the kitchen is less abstract.

- Other factors that may affect someone's ability in making choices from day to day that should be taken into consideration might be health, mood, interest, or how tired they are.

- Consider the number of choices offered to a person as this can also affect their ability to make a choice.

- Don't forget to involve people in small choices such as which bow to decorate a present with.

- Consider breaking down a larger decision into smaller parts, such as choosing different elements to build up a picture of how a person wants to decorate their room.

- When supporting someone to make a choice, it is important to check that what you think they are saying is actually the choice they are making. Sometimes people are able to make clear choices, for example pointing or reaching for something or clearly expressing a choice verbally. At other times the choice that someone makes may be less clear, for example by facial expression.

- Consider asking for confirmation from a person or presenting the choice in a different way to ensure that you understand what they want.

- It is common for people to choose the last thing that is offered to them. If this is a possibility, it can be useful to present the same choice in a different order to check the validity of that choice for the person.

- A person's experience of the options (how informed that choice is) can affect how they make choices. When supporting a person to make choices and decisions, it is therefore important to give them the opportunity to explore and experience different options so they can make a comparison.

Examples of methods of supporting people to make choices include:

- thumbs up and thumbs down

- happy and sad faces

- choice boards

- key-rings

- pointing

- using pictures, symbols and photographs to make choices accessible, eg menus, activities

- supporting informed choice by making information accessible around the subject

- collecting views and opinions through collages, scrapbooks or posters

- giving people experiences or tasters of options and gaining feedback by using these communication methods or by observing responses.

## Reflection

Consider some of the ways in which you involve people with a learning disability in choice and decision making.

Some people with more complex needs may be supported to show preference rather than make a choice as such (Ware, 2004a). Preference can be shown even when someone does not intentionally communicate. The person may not necessarily have a cognitive conception or memory of what the choice options are. Understanding preference involves observing reactions and responses to one stimulus at a time. Over time, preferences can be established if a person's response to something is consistent. Time should be taken to explore someone's reactions to different stimuli. For example, you might observe that someone consistently shows that they enjoy time in the sensory room or that they do not like the taste of fish.

When offering new stimuli or activities, it is important not to assume that someone is making a choice if they initially push something away or refuse to engage in something. It may be that the person needs more time or experience to get used to the new stimulus or activity.

To understand someone's preferences, people need to be given the opportunity to explore a range of experiences. Sensitive and considered support is ethically important as every attempt should be made to give people increased choice and control over their lives. Understanding how someone shows preference can enable this, even if they are unable to make choices in the more conventional sense.

At times, decisions may need to be made on behalf of people who lack capacity, especially people who have more complex communication or cognitive needs. Where people lack the capacity to make a decision independently, the Mental Capacity Act 2005 outlines how decisions are made in someone's 'best interests'. Such decisions are generally made by people who know the person best and may involve a meeting or discussions with family, friends, an advocate, paid support staff and other professionals. For people who do not have an independent person involved, Independent Mental Capacity Advocates (IMCA) are available to independently support decision-making in the person's best interests. Although the person may lack the capacity to be supported to make a final choice themselves, there may be elements of that decision that the individual will be able to be involved in that will influence the decision. See Toby's example at the end of this section.

A decision should only be made on someone's behalf when all methods of supporting them to make a choice have been exhausted. Person-centred frameworks and non-directive advocacy approaches are examples of how practitioners may consider making decisions on behalf of a person.

## Person-centred approaches

Taking a person-centred approach is about focusing on what we believe is important to the person. This can be determined by:

- getting to know a person through building a relationship with them over time

- building a picture of the person with other people who know them really well

- observing preferences and personality

- discussing how a person communicates and indicates preferences with people who know them well

- checking interpretations and not making assumptions

- using existing documents to develop a picture of the person's life.

## Watching Brief

The Watching Brief was developed by Assist (an advocacy project in Staffordshire, UK) in 1994. The method provides a useful framework to support people who are making a decision on someone else's behalf. It proposes eight domains to a quality of life and helps practitioners to structure questions that could help make a decision. These are how the decision might affect:

- **a person's competence**

- **community presence**

- **choice and influence**

- **continuity**

- **status and respect**

- **individuality**

- **well-being**

- **partnerships and relationships.**

(Voices through Advocacy, 2008)

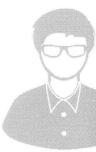

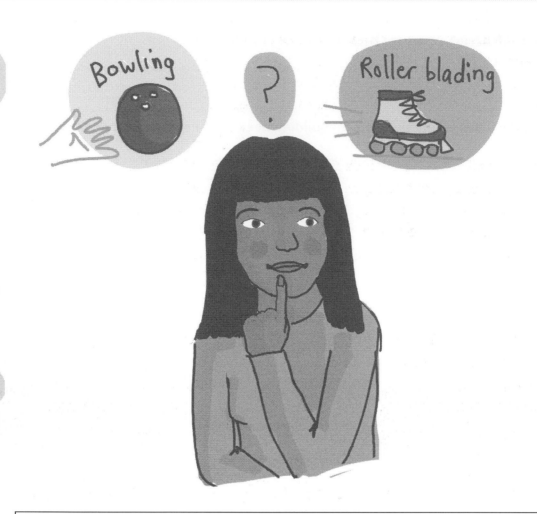

## Examples of good practice

### Making choices

At the local college, students in the catering department worked with students from the department supporting people with a learning disability to make an accessible menu for the refectory. The students took photographs of all the menu options, including drinks and snacks. Menus were compiled using the photographs with text indicating the name, description and price of each option. The 'choice of the day' board was also redesigned so that there was space next to each option for a photograph. Each month, as part of their menu-planning classes, the catering students worked alongside the students with learning disability to update the accessible menu. To make menu choices, some students are supported by their support worker at the table to look through the menu to make their choices;

other students like to queue up and place their own order with the catering students working in the refectory, who are shown how to support people to make menu choices.

Kelly is supported to choose what to wear each morning. Because choice between too many options is overwhelming for Kelly, her support worker takes

Speechmark

out a small selection of clothes from her wardrobe that are suitable for the weather that day.

The options are laid on the bed for Kelly to look at. When Kelly's support worker touches the item that Kelly wants, her face lights up and she becomes more vocal.

Bushra has a bag of objects of reference that she has built up with her community support worker. Each object represents an activity that she enjoys doing during the morning they spend together each week. Before they go out, Bushra is supported to select an object; objects that represent activities that are unsuitable on that morning (for example due to weather) are removed beforehand.

## Informed choices or decisions

Inga and Vicky are saving up to have their bedrooms redecorated. Previously, when they have had their rooms decorated, the staff who know them really well have led the decision making by choosing what they think Inga and Vicky would like, based on their knowledge of them and their tastes. Their support staff want them to be more involved in the decision making. To achieve this, they put two large sheets of paper on the wall and wrote 'Inga's room' on one and 'Vicky's room' on the other. Over a few weeks, the whole team supported Vicky and Inga to collect magazines, catalogues and samples of wallpaper and carpet. In the evenings, they were supported to look through them. Anything they liked, regardless of price, was cut out and the girls stuck these onto the paper to make a collage.

As the weeks passed, very distinct themes could be seen on the collages – Inga loved pinks, soft floral designs, feathers and diamanté. Vicky chose greens and blues, and she loved chandeliers, regal-looking furniture and gilded frames. Vicky's choices were very different from the way her room was previously decorated. Once the collages were complete, Inga and Vicky were supported to convert their dream rooms into real choices by sourcing items that matched their taste within their budget. At the next team meeting, the team agreed that they were surprised by the strong contrast between the two collages and the very definite themes that emerged in each collage. Even though Vicky and Inga couldn't describe what they wanted in words, and some staff members felt that Vicky especially couldn't make consistent choices, the collage that they had each created demonstrated very clearly their individuality and their choices.

Toby leaves school at the end of the year. Meetings have been held including Toby, his social worker, teachers and family to discuss what Toby would like to do after leaving school. Although Toby does not communicate verbally, he is fully involved in this choice. Over the last few months, Toby has been supported to visit various options available to him in the local area and has built up a scrapbook of what he likes or dislikes about these options. Some were indicated by Toby (for example, that the access into and around the college in his wheelchair was good and got a thumbs up) and some were inferred by his reaction to the experience (for example, he became very anxious at one day service he visited which was very noisy because there were a lot of people in large areas for much of the time). He was also supported to build a portfolio of what he liked doing and what made him happy. People who knew Toby well were at the meeting and were able to add other information such as the level of support he would need and the cost implications of transport. Although Toby was considered not to have the capacity to make this decision independently, he was supported to be fully involved in the decision making at his Best Interests meetings.

Maud was in hospital for surgery to remove a cyst on her fallopian tubes. This was the second time she had been admitted for the planned surgery. On the first occasion, the surgeon refused to carry out the procedure because he didn't believe that Maud had the capacity to consent to the surgery and her support staff were not able to give consent on her behalf. Maud's support staff had spent a lot of time with her explaining about the cyst, what the surgery involved and what the risks were and felt that Maud was able to give informed consent. Following the first appointment, the support worker took a copy of the consent paper and wrote a version that was accessible to Maud using simple language, pictures and symbols. This copy was attached to the hospital consent form and accepted by the surgeon as consent to the procedure on the second occasion along with a discussion with Maud about the procedure.

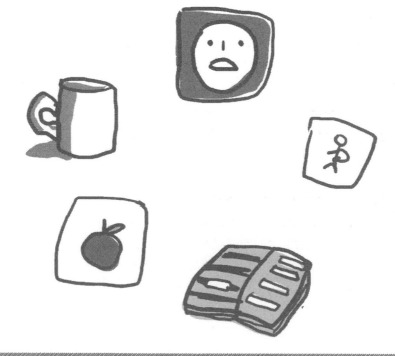

# Supporting people to explore and express themselves

Throughout our lives we have opportunities to consider and develop who we are and what is important to us: by meeting different people; being exposed to different ideas and ways of thinking; challenging how we perceive the world through learning; and by experiencing different activities and roles in life. This is a lifelong learning journey and people continually develop and change as individuals. What is important to a teenager and how this is expressed through fashion, activities and language may be different from that is important to the same person 10, 20 or 30 years later.

People with a learning disability are likely to have more limited opportunities to explore and develop who they are and what is important to them. Communication partners can offer them opportunities to do this through, for example:

- Providing varied activities, experiences and opportunities to do different things.

- Giving them opportunities to explore issues, consider current affairs and understand news items.

- Learning about their own and other people's culture, religion, food and drink, fashion and music.

- Finding out about what other people like about them, what they are good at and what they think is important to them (and whether they agree).

- Providing opportunities to have different roles and responsibilities.

- Developing existing interests and introducing similar interests to those they already have.

- Offering a safe, non-judgemental environment in which they can explore, experience and express.

It is important to consider how to support people with a learning disability to access these opportunities, particularly those who use alternative methods of communication.

This may be achieved through experiential learning by engaging in activities, themed days or projects where people can experience sensory aspects of other cultures, or experience different roles and responsibilities. Supporting people to engage in more abstract opportunities (such as current affairs, news items, and other issues that may be relevant or of interest) can be achieved by using story boards, role play, drama, film, or art through drawing or modelling.

Self-expression is about portraying yourself to others. When we consider the methods that we use to portray ourselves to others (such as how we dress, the activities we choose to do, the roles we choose in society and the values and opinions we have), the barriers which may be faced by many people with a learning disability start to become evident. We need to consider how they too can be supported in these areas.

The ways in which people are supported to do everyday tasks and activities can either help people overcome these barriers or they can contribute to barriers preventing self-expression. Skills in enabling choice and supporting people to express an opinion are fundamental to being part of overcoming these barriers.

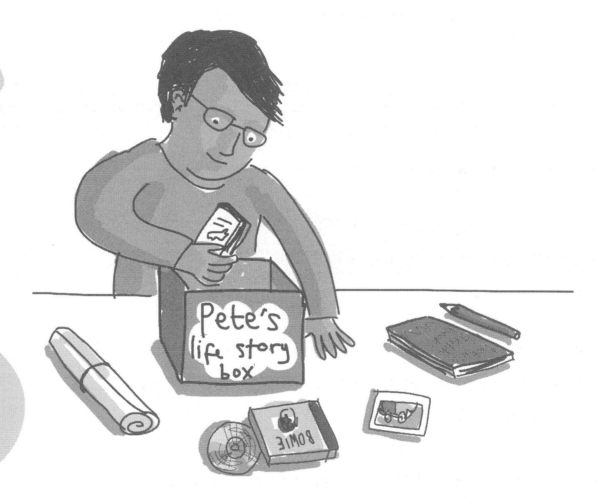

Supporting self-expression may be achieved through:

- Supporting people to make choices; even simple ones between two options such as which T-shirt to wear.

- Giving people opportunities to express themselves.

Speechmark

- Taking time to get to know how a person communicates.

- Learning to understand how people express preference, choice and whether they like or dislike something; for example, through facial expressions, gestures and sounds.

- Giving people the tools to express preference, choice and whether they like or dislike something; for example, through signing, pointing to an object or symbols that demonstrate opinion and using technology such as BIGmack™ buttons.

- Actively seeking opinions.

- Supporting the person to do things for themselves, rather than doing them for the person.

- Making time to support people to be more involved and have more independence.

- Making time to 'listen' to people.

- Not assuming that people have no opinion or have 'nothing to say' just because they don't communicate this verbally.

There are also activities that can be used to support people to explore and express themselves. These include:

- Organising person-centred planning activities.

- Making collages of items that interest them or are important to them.

- Building up a photograph album of activities and experiences that they have enjoyed.

- Having sessions to try different styles of clothes, make-up, hairstyles, etc.

- Making a story board or poster about a news item or historical event.

- Making a film or video.

- Creating an animation.

- Creating a personal box with objects of reference and photos of activities, people and places that are important to the person.

- Creating an online communication passport or a presentation using software such as PowerPoint.

- A scrapbook of activities that have been tried and places that have been visited.

- An identity mirror: pictures, symbols and words that represent the person, their interests and personality are fixed around the mirror.

## Reflection

1  Consider the following questions about yourself.

   • Who am I?

   • What is important to me?

   • What are my dreams or nightmares?

   • What are my gifts? What am I good at?

2  On a piece of paper, represent your thoughts and ideas using words, pictures or graphics.

(*Source*: based on MAPS – see O'Brien et al, 2010)

## Examples of good practice

A day service introduced a weekly theme. Some of the themes were suggested by service users, others were in response to news or calendar events. Examples of these themes included:

• Chinese New Year

• Friendship

• Spring

• An earthquake in Japan

• France and French culture

• The weather

• Farm animals

• The Royal Wedding

• The Olympics

• The Government and voting.

These themes were reflected in the sessions during the week. At the entrance to the building, two large boards displayed work around the themes; one was a work in progress built up of photographs and items made during that week. The other was the previous week's completed theme.

A community support worker supported an older man to build up a portfolio of photographs, souvenirs and drawings, showing the places where he liked to go and what he liked about each place.

Violet was supported to write her own person-centred plans to help staff get to know her and how she liked to be supported; the first part of her plan was all about 'who I am and what is important to me'. People who knew her well such as family, friends, her favourite teacher at school, and one of her support staff also contributed with suggestions. Violet collected photographs, drew pictures and used symbols alongside the text.

Emily has severe learning disabilities. Her family helped her to make a personal life box which contained objects and photographs that were important to her. The life box helped her to remember some of her experiences, such as holidays and family parties. Emily's family attached labels with information about the objects and pictures so that people who worked with her could talk to her about them.

A college which supports students with learning disabilities helped Jonathan to make a multimedia presentation about what was important to him. He then showed his presentation to his friends and to other people he met, which helped him to talk about himself, his interests and his feelings. The multimedia presentation used video clips of Jonathan doing his favourite things, music he liked, sound effects and graphics. Jonathan was involved in choosing the media items and deciding how they were put together.

# Activity planning

People with a learning disability can be excluded from being involved in planning because of some of the difficulties that this may present. Decisions such as where to go for lunch, or what to do on Saturday afternoon, or what to do after school next year may be made on behalf of these people. Communication partners can support them to be more involved in activity planning in both the short and the long term.

A person's ability to be involved in planning activities may range from choosing between two or more options, being involved in the content and details of an activity or contributing new ideas and suggestions.

Some people with learning disabilities have not had experience of being, or opportunities to be, involved in planning, so it is important to consider where opportunities exist and to develop skills and confidence in planning.

The following tools may be used to support planning.

- Choice boards (see page 149)

- Objects of reference (see page 84)

- Photographs of choice options: for example, places to go, things to do.

- Key-rings with different options on them (see page 81).

- Timetables with spaces to add choices (see page 77).

- Posters of preferences to build up a picture of what a person enjoys or would like.

- Dream catchers – hanging ideas and dreams for the future represented in ways that the person can understand.

- Person-centred planning approaches (see page 132).

- Gathering ideas from people who know the person best and using these as options.

- Using past experience and knowledge of what the person has enjoyed, or has worked well in the past, and using these as options.

- Creating a weekly schedule to help review what people currently do and what they would like to do by selecting symbols or pictures, as appropriate.

- Drawing what the activity (eg a weekend away) would look like, who would be there, how we would travel, etc.

- Using graphic facilitation to collect ideas from a group (see page 141)

Planning involves thinking about what is going to happen in the future, whether this is after lunch, the day after tomorrow or next month. Most people with a learning disability find the concept of time confusing, so it is as important to support a person to understand when the outcome of a choice is going to happen as it is to make the choice itself. Offering a choice about something that is going to happen in the future without understanding when this is going to happen can cause anxiety and frustration and, in some cases, lead to behaviours that can be challenging.

Visual representations can help people to understand the passage of time. By including information such as fixed events, or routines that are known and familiar to the person, they can be supported to place an event in time. People may have an understanding of the rhythms and routines of familiar events even if they don't fully understand the terms we use for their frequency. For example, going swimming weekly; visiting Gran and Granddad monthly; birthdays and Christmas are once a year. Supporting someone to understand that a planned activity is going take place 'on the same day that we go swimming', 'the weekend after we next see Gran and Granddad' or 'after Christmas' adds meaning.

Examples of visual representations of time include:

- A plan for the day showing fixed activities such as breakfast, lunch and tea as points of reference.

- A table showing today and tomorrow and including other known activities.

- Timetables for the days of the week. Days may be identified by association with other information such as school, favourite soaps on television, going out with Dad on Saturday.

- A countdown of the number of 'sleeps' before an event.

- A time line showing other key events such as birthdays, Christmas, school holidays, etc.

- Calendars where the days are crossed off or a pointer is moved.

Supporting people with more complex learning disabilities to be involved in short- and long-term planning is more challenging as this group of people may experience difficulties in understanding cause and effect (making a choice and relating this to the ensuing activity). They may also have little understanding of time and routines, have limited memory, and present more challenges in supporting communication.

People with more complex disabilities also typically have the least experience and skills in making plans. However, it is just as important to offer opportunities to be involved in making plans for the future. To facilitate involvement in making meaningful plans, an activity should begin immediately after supporting the person to make a choice so that the cause and effect of the action taken is reinforced. When supporting choice-making with this group, there is often a greater role for sensitive advocacy.

To support learning, opportunities to make plans need to be frequent and presented consistently in the same way. Involvement in planning for activities that will take place in the future, whether tomorrow or in six months' time, is also possible. However, it may instead focus on identifying a person's preferences, previous experiences which have been enjoyable, and learning from what has worked or not worked for the person in the past.

## Reflection

Sarah and Laura are two young women who need pictorial support to make choices and decisions as they find abstract choices difficult.

Consider how you would support them to plan for their holiday.

## Examples of good practice

Going out in the car for a cup of tea each day was identified as the most important part of Charlotte's day when she made her own person-centred plan. When her support staff were asked who decides where Charlotte goes, they realised that each of them had their own list of places to go and would make a choice based on the weather that day or the time they had available. After further discussion, the team decided to support Charlotte to choose where to go herself.

With Charlotte, the staff took photographs of all the places that she enjoyed going to and laminated them. On the back of the photographs there were directions to the venue and information such as 'not suitable in wet weather', 'needs at least two hours', 'no café, take a flask'. Initially, they used a small selection of photographs to support Charlotte to point to her preference. Over the weeks, she began to be able to choose between an increasing number of options until she could look through the whole box until she found the photograph she wanted. Staff continued to add new options and introduced a photograph of Charlotte using the camera to let her know that they were going to a new place.

**Speechmark**

Knowing what was going to happen each day was really important to Samir. Not knowing caused him great anxiety which could lead to self-harm and aggressive outbursts towards other people. Samir used a visual timetable which he helped staff to update each week. This was used to support him to talk about what he was going to do or what he had done that day. Some activities were fixed; for example, school during the week and youth club on a Friday evening. Some activities were chosen by him in advance, such as what he wanted to do in the evenings (eg jigsaws, baking, drawing). Other activities such as 'going out with Mum and Dad' were put on the timetable but the details were decided on the day. The symbols for the activities he enjoyed were stuck to the bottom of the timetable for Samir to move into place.

Sarah and Laura were supported to plan their holiday by building up a scrapbook of wishes, including whether they would consider flying, or going by coach or train; the activities they would like to do while on holiday; how long they wanted to go for; whether they wanted to be in the city, countryside, by the sea, etc. The support staff then looked at a range of holiday options within their price range. They put together an A3-sized poster for each option which showed aspects of the holiday, including pictures of the accommodation, symbols for the mode of transport and symbols or pictures for the activities available. Sarah and Laura used the posters to consider and choose which holiday they preferred.

When Harry's support staff began to discuss why they supported him to engage in certain activities, they realised that they made choices based on their experience of his responses to activities in the past. They knew that Harry enjoyed being outdoors if it was sunny, even if it was cold; that he became more vocal and animated when music was played; that he loved water (baths, the hydrotherapy pool and putting his hands or feet in water); that lights and gentle music relaxed him and that he didn't like noise from too many people or from the television.

Even though Harry's team had supported him for many years, they had never formally discussed how they knew what he liked and disliked. This was recorded in his plans along with activities or aspects of activities that they knew he enjoyed. To support Harry to start making choices between activities, the team introduced different object cues (an actual object that was used in the activity) which were given to Harry to hold before and during an activity. After several weeks, Harry's staff team started to notice that Harry began to become more animated when given objects related to activities that he liked. They are hoping that, over time, Harry will be able to show a preference between two activities by his response to actual objects that are given to him.

Narinder was supported to take part in short-term activity planning by being told a story about someone who went to the cinema. Narinder's support worker made up a story which included travelling to the cinema, buying a ticket and how much it cost, buying snacks, what it was like in the auditorium (lighting level, how loud it was, how many other people were there), what the film was like and how long it lasted. The support worker also used objects (eg cinema ticket, brochure, popcorn bag) and relevant photographs (the bus stop, the cinema, promotional photographs for the film, etc). Narinder was encouraged to ask questions during the story and to make suggestions about what might happen next. This helped Narinder to understand the activity more fully and to make choices about whether and how she wanted to participate in the activity.

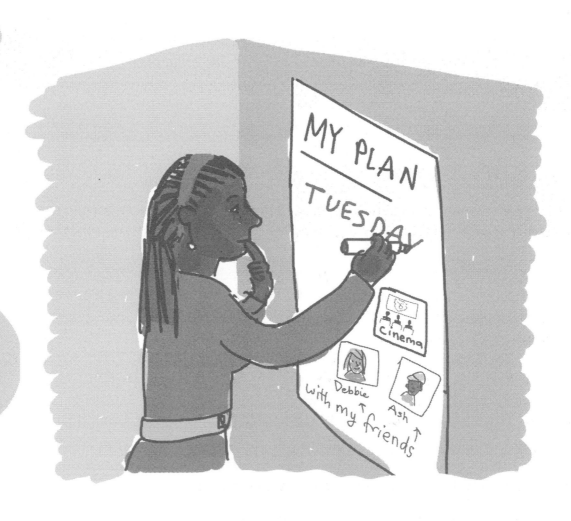

# Consultation around communication

It is good practice to regularly review communication when working with people with a learning disability. It provides an opportunity to consider what is working and what is not working; it refreshes people's work practice to ensure that methods that have been shown to be successful continue to be used and new practices and any changes in support needs are shared.

Consulting with others about communication shows a commitment to working in partnership with people and promoting opportunities to listen and share knowledge and experiences. Opportunities to share knowledge about how someone communicates are valuable and can make an enormous difference to the way in which someone is supported.

Continuity between the ways in which different people work with a person is as important with regard to communication as it is with any other support needs. Discussions about communication approaches and how a person communicates should feature on agendas at reviews and meetings.

As communication does not tend to feature on agendas in multidisciplinary reviews or meetings, it is often surprising what is revealed when it is (see the example of Manchu later). It is important that information around changing communication needs and methods are recorded, updated and shared regularly.

## Reflection

Consider some of the ways in which you consult about communication.

Who is involved in this process?

Involving people in consultation about how they prefer to communicate may involve:

- Observing how the person chooses to communicate.

- Observing the person's body language and emotions.

- Observing their reaction to different communication methods. Do they appear to be uninterested, frustrated or confused or are they more interested and focused?

- Reflecting on what appears to be working or not working in how you communicate.

- Checking with the person using a simple 'yes/no' system (thumbs up or down, or smiley and sad faces) or signing, if they can convey their opinions in this way.

- Using Talking Mats™ to gauge how a person feels about the communication approach or system and pictorially ranking them.

- Sharing information with people who know the person well both within the team and with family, friends, advocates and support staff from other services.

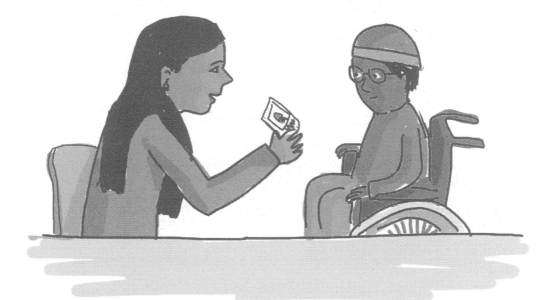

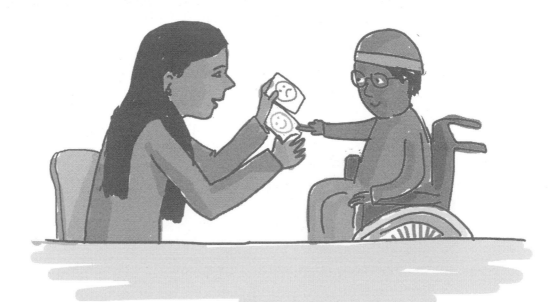

## Examples of good practice

When students start at a college for young adults with learning disabilities, a questionnaire is sent to the student, their family and/or home to collect information about the student's support needs, including communication. A meeting is arranged twice a year with the student and key people to discuss learning. Part of this meeting focuses on how the student communicates, including any new methods and tools that have been used, or new signs and symbols that have been learned. These meetings are an opportunity to learn more about how the student communicates at home and to discuss how learning at college can be transferred to other areas of the student's life. The college also encourages students to use a communication book which travels to and from the college with the student. Among other issues, the book is used to record developments in communication such as new signs learned that week.

During an activity carried out by a speech and language therapist, Manchu showed that he could match pictures with simple words. During his review, Manchu's support staff at home were amazed as none of them were aware that Manchu could do this. This information was then used to re-evaluate the communication opportunities offered to Manchu.

Nicole moved from children's services to adults' services two years ago. She is now settled in her new home and appears relaxed and happy with her support staff and co-tenant. She has some verbal communication but appears quiet and shy much of the time, choosing to engage in solitary activities or enjoying watching other activities in the house. As part of her review, the manager of Nicole's staff team visited Nicole at college and at the club she attended on a Friday night. At the college, he discovered that Nicole could recognise a much larger vocabulary of signs and was better at signing back than he had realised; at the club, he was able to share how Nicole could be supported to choose between activities by using flash cards with pictures of different options.

When he met with the family at the review meeting, it transpired that family members also used some signs but admitted that they didn't always understand some of the signs that Nicole used with them. A training session was arranged for the support staff at Nicole's home to refresh their knowledge of signs and symbols and to learn new ones and Nicole's family was invited to attend.

Laurence has profound and multiple learning disabilities. The teacher and teaching assistants did not always understand what his behaviour communicated (vocalisations, facial expressions, gestures, whole body movements, rate of breathing, etc). With the permission of Laurence's parents, they filmed short sections of his day. The staff and the family watched the videos and they each made observations of what they thought he might be communicating. Together, they wrote a list of what they thought certain behaviours may be communicating and they all met again six weeks later to discuss whether their first thoughts seemed to be accurate.

Speechmark

# Consultation around making information accessible

The key to producing accessible information that can be understood by people with learning disabilities is to consult with the people for whom it is being made accessible. In the absence of consultation, there is a risk that the information is no more accessible than printed information and that the exercise is tokenistic.

People with learning disabilities can be involved in making information accessible by deciding on the format in which it is presented and its content, including wording and the pictures or symbols used to make the information easier to understand.

Consultation may also take place by people with learning disabilities looking over documents to check that the information is accessible to them and giving feedback about what works and what doesn't work before the final version is produced.

If the information being made accessible is for an individual or a small group, consultation may take place with the whole target audience. If the target audience is much larger (eg for a newsletter or accessible policies), consultation may take place with a sample of the target audience. When setting up a consultation group, it is important to include people who use a range of communication methods. There are also locally established groups of people with a learning disability who regularly give feedback on information made accessible by services. Because these people are independent, they may feel more able to say that they cannot fully understand the information produced if this is the case.

It is important to consider that accessible information produced for people with a learning disability to understand may still rely on the support of a communication partner to interpret it. While a person is supported to understand accessible information, the communication partner can use this as a way of checking if the methods used are appropriate to the person and that they can understand it. If the person carrying out the consultation is not a regular communication partner with a person, it is important to involve other people who know that person well (family, support worker, teacher) in facilitating consultation around communication.

In the same way that, when learning to read text, an ability to read the words does not mean that a person understands what is being communicated through those words, a person with a learning disability may be able to understand individual pictures or symbols but not understand what is being communicated. A communication partner's role may also need to be to help the person understand the meaning of material that is made accessible. This can be achieved by giving examples relating to the person's life and helping them to engage with the material on a personal level. Checking a person's understanding of the material can also be a way to check whether the methods used are a good way of communicating with that person.

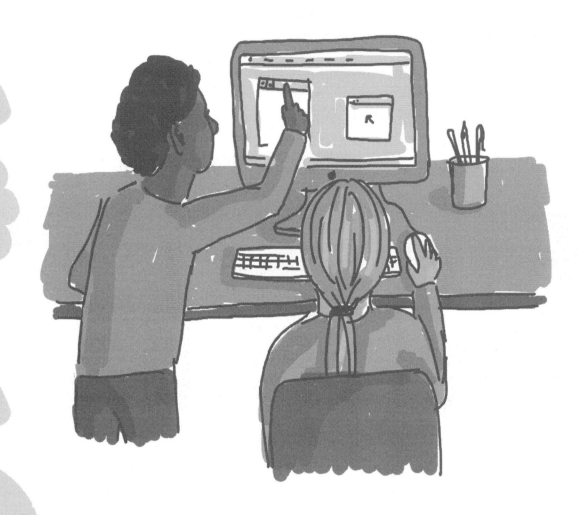

## Reflection

In your work practice, consider what information could be made accessible to the people you support.

- How could you make this accessible?

- How would you involve the people you support?

Speechmark

## Examples of good practice

When producing documents such as the service user guide, a day service supporting people with learning disabilities invited a group of service users with different communication needs to approve or amend the way the document was made accessible before it was finalised.

An organisation which provides supported accommodation for adults with a learning disability involved a group of service users in managing the production of a newsletter. Members of the team were supported to carry out all the tasks, including collecting information, putting the newsletter together, making the information accessible, taking photographs for articles or upcoming events and distributing the finished product.

A community support group periodically sent out letters and information about new groups or activities in the local area that people may be interested in. Although addressed to the people who accessed the service, the information was not necessarily accessible to them because it was assumed that the information would be conveyed by parents, carers or support staff.

They have recently started to send out letters and information in an accessible format. Before doing so, they consulted with a sample group of service users about the ways in which information could best be made accessible for them. The group was supported to put together some guidelines that would be followed each time information was produced for sending out. Because information was sent out regularly and, at times, only a short while before the events took place, the group continued to meet at regular intervals for several months to give feedback on information, rather than checking information before it was sent out. Suggestions for improvement were then added to the guidelines.

# Involving people in meetings and reviews

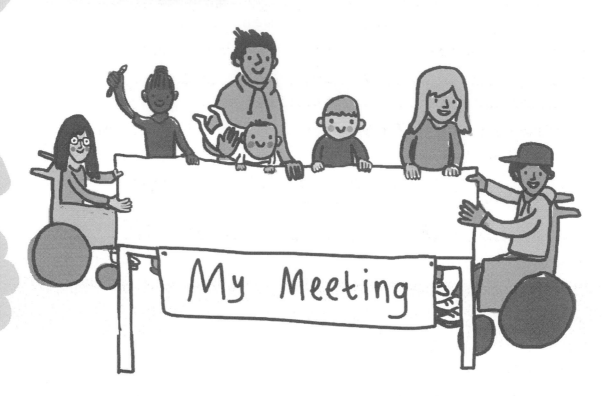

Services that support people with learning disabilities should regularly have meetings and reviews with the people they support. These are important forums for making decisions, recording progress, agreeing action plans, flagging up problems and concerns, planning for the future and celebrating success.

Traditionally, reviews and meetings were led by professionals who prepared the agenda and frequently used a service pro forma. Records were held by professionals, included in the person's file (which was accessed by professionals) and circulated to others involved in the person's life. It was not uncommon for meetings and reviews to take place in the absence of family, advocates or even the person involved. There has been tremendous progress towards including and involving people with learning disabilities in meetings and reviews about them.

Meetings and reviews involving people with a learning disability need to be tailored to the needs of the individual. This might include how a person communicates, how they can be involved in the process, how they like to participate, and their level of concentration and interest. A standardised format or process for conducting meetings and reviews may not work for everyone. Involving people in meetings and reviews about them, in a meaningful way, influences the outcome of the decisions that are made and ensures that their views and wishes are heard.

It might be useful to consider the following factors when planning a meeting or review. Before the meeting or review, consider:

- Does everybody know how the person communicates and how best to communicate with them in their preferred way? Consider making communication passports, communication dictionaries, or other records of how the person prefers to communicate, available to the people involved in the meeting.

- Making time in advance of the meeting for the individual to contribute to the agenda and think about what he or she wants to discuss.

- Producing an agenda which is accessible to the person and includes issues contributed by them.

- Helping the person to gather and understand information about issues that are going to be talked about before the meeting.

- Using photos to support a person to decide who they want to come to a review or to show the person who is coming to a review.

- Offering the person an advocate to support them.

- Talking through key issues with the person before the meeting.

- Supporting people to consider and make decisions before meetings, at their own pace.

During the meeting or review, consider:

- Including the person in the meeting! Does the person want to be involved?

- Involving other people who know the person well – family, advocate, support staff, key people from other services accessed by the person (in consultation with the individual).

- Using communication methods such as talking mats, symbols or signing.

- Showing videos and photographs of the person (make sure that the person feels comfortable with this or consents to it).

- Ensuring that any communication tools are taken into the review that may be needed to support someone to communicate about what they want and feel is important or to express feelings.

- What makes the person feel calm or relaxed in a meeting?

- Would it be helpful to split the meeting into small chunks, take rest breaks, or provide refreshments, or would this be a distraction?

- Making information accessible throughout the meeting through methods such as graphic facilitation, using simple language, using easy words and checking that the person understands.

- The language you use is important. Try not to use jargon; if it is used, help people to understand it.

- Using egg-timers to help people not to talk for too long, if this might affect concentration.

- Using sensory stories to support the person to understand the context and to express preferences.

- Using stories to help the person to tell others what they do and what is important to them or to explain situations.

- Using activities to explore how people might be feeling.

- Using person-centred planning approaches and referring to communication passports, portfolios and objects of significance that a person may bring in to show people.

- How a person's views are represented if they find it difficult to make their own wishes, needs or views known.

After the meeting, consider:

- How meetings are recorded – are minutes made accessible to the individual? Have they got their own copy?

- Whether minutes are checked with the individual to make sure that they represent what was said and agreed.

- How a person is supported to know that they have a right to complain.

- If decisions were made that the person is not happy with, how is this explained to them or how are they supported to redress this?

- How the person responded to the process and record this if appropriate. What was learned? What worked or didn't work?

- How the process could be improved. How could the person be involved more effectively?

## Reflection

- How do you involve people with learning disabilities in meetings or reviews if this is applicable to your role or work practice?

- What changes or improvements could be made to enable some of the people you work with to take part in the meeting or review?

Speechmark

## Examples of good practice

A school for children and young people with learning disabilities have regular meetings to discuss and review learning. The meeting includes the student, their parents or carers, the teacher and sometimes a classroom assistant or other professionals who may be involved, such as a speech and language therapist.

In preparation for the meeting, the teacher collects examples of work the student has done. He sends home an accessible agenda (the pro forma which was made accessible with students from the school) for the parent or carer to support the student to look at and add their own comments in the space provided. This pro forma and the work done by the student in class is used to support the student to focus on and be involved in the discussions. A summary using pictures, symbols and easy words is then sent home with a more detailed report.

Rebecca's community support worker reviews the work she does with Rebecca every six months. This ensures that any changing support needs are recorded and any issues arising are addressed. It also gives Rebecca an opportunity to reflect on what she has enjoyed and what else she might like to do in the next six months. Rebecca is sent a letter with a few questions so that her Mum can support Rebecca to plan for the review. During the review, photographs of activities Rebecca has been involved in are used to help her think about what she has enjoyed and what has worked or not worked. On a large sheet of paper on the table, Rebecca's support worker draws a person in the middle with 'Rebecca' written underneath and arrows to a smiley face (where things that Rebecca has enjoyed or have worked are written or drawn); and a sad face (where things that Rebecca didn't enjoy or didn't work are written or drawn). Another arrow points to a drawing of Rebecca and her community support worker (where changes in her support needs are written or drawn). The bottom half of the page has a road drawn on it with a signpost pointing from left to right. Along the road are written or drawn any agreed actions or plans for the future.

Maureen's community support worker noticed how, during a review meeting, she became withdrawn and upset. Maureen was supported to think about things that made her happy and sad by collecting objects and pictures which she turned into a collage to help her communicate with other people.

James was supported to take part in his review by his support worker who made a story about some of his activities and how he takes part in them. James' support worker used simple speech, objects and pictures to help James tell his story to other people (based on Storysharing® by Nicola Grove).

Clare's mother made some short films which showed her child's facial expressions and reactions to things that made her happy and sad. These video clips helped people in the review to think about Clare's responses to different support she accessed.

# Understanding change

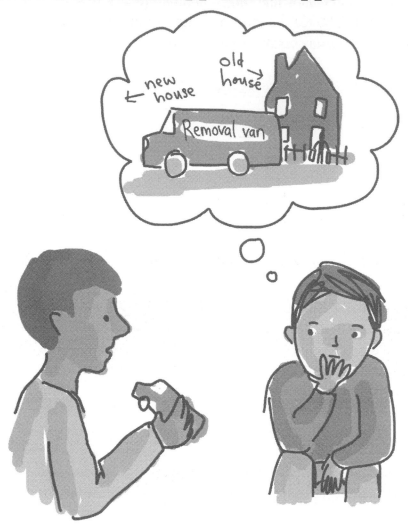

Familiarity and routine make life more predictable and can help people feel in control of their environment and experience. When change occurs, the amount of information that needs to be processed is greatly increased and people with learning disability may experience difficulties in this area. The consequences of change are also difficult for people to understand and so the full impact of a change may not be apparent until some time after the change has occurred.

When changes occur that are unexpected, not understood or not prepared for, that change can have a significant impact on a person with a learning disability, especially if they are autistic or have autistic traits. Change can cause uncertainty, distress, anxiety, confusion, fear, insecurity and feelings of being out of control. People may also struggle to know what is expected of them. These feelings are most frequently expressed by changes in behaviour at the time of the change or some time after the change has occurred, when the consequences of the change are experienced.

**Speechmark**

Supporting people to understand change can be an important part of managing behaviours and helping a person feel safe and secure. Supporting people to prepare for change, where this can be anticipated, can help lessen the impact and support people to feel more comfortable with change. Support during and after change is also important, particularly when events cannot be anticipated.

Some examples of changes that may require support include:

- Changes in timetabled or planned activity.

- Changes in the days or times when a service is attended.

- Changes in support staff – a permanent or temporary change due to sickness, holiday, etc. This may be planned or unplanned.

- Changes in day service routine due to holiday, bank holiday, weather conditions.

- Changes in the day or time of a favourite television programme.

- Changes in transport arrangements.

- Changes in environment – redecorating, changing furniture around, building work, etc.

- Clocks going forward or back one hour.

- Transition between services, eg leaving school or college, changing a day service.

- Moving house.

- Going on holiday.

- New co-tenant, group or class member.

- Adolescence – emotional, physical and social changes.

- Personal ill health which results in short- or long-term changes in activity, routine or environment.

- Bereavement or ill health of a family member or friend – and the changes that this may involve for the person.

## Reflection

Think of examples of when you might support people through change.

- How might the person feel if they are not helped to understand change?

- How could you involve the person in anticipating and dealing with that change?

The strategies that can be used to support people through change include:

- Anticipating change. What is involved in the change, when is the change planned or likely to happen?

- Preparing people in advance where possible.

- Offering familiarity and stability through other areas of the person's life; other planned changes in the person's life may be postponed.

- Using clear, simple, precise language that is unambiguous and concrete.

- Repetition – the same information may need to be repeated many times in the same way or in different ways to support the person to understand the change.

- Allowing time for the person to process information.

- Considering how much detail is given – there must be enough information to enable understanding; however, too much detail can be overwhelming.

- Considering how a person is supported to understand the whole process, not just the end result (eg. going on holiday will require an understanding of packing, the mode of travel, sleeping somewhere new, different routines while away, different food, etc).

- Considering how a person is supported to understand when the change is going to happen (see the information in the section on activity planning).

- Considering how a person is supported to feel in control of the change as much as possible by involving them in the process and the decision-making.

- Considering how a person is supported to understand what their role will be and what is expected of them.

- Considering how a person is supported to become familiar with a new situation: for example, by visiting the new classroom, school, house, day service; meeting the new support worker, teacher, etc.

Speechmark

- Working with other people who may be involved, sharing knowledge and understanding of the person: for example, how they can be supported when anxious during or after change.

- Sharing information around communication methods so that the person can be more effectively supported in different situations, or by different people.

- How you support someone to understand the emotional consequence of change. This requires sensitivity around someone's response to understanding change.

The methods to achieve this might include:

- Making a scrapbook about the upcoming change – eg a holiday, new experience, new service.

- Drawing

- Role play

- Use 'now' and 'next' boards that use photos or symbols or objects to support people through the process of change. This can be helpful to reduce anxiety even if a person can usually process more information.

- Use storytelling, film or a story board to help a person understand the change.

- Using memory books or boxes or photo albums to celebrate the past or come to terms with loss.

- Use visual support such as graphic facilitation, pictures, symbols or visual timetables to explain change.

- Accessing specialist learning disability counselling.

### Examples of good practice

When May was supported to choose where she lived after living with family all her life, she was supported to visit a range of options: seeing the location of the property in relation to bus routes, local shops and the other services she accessed; viewing the bedroom she would have; and meeting the people she would live with and the staff who would support her. She had regular meal time visits and sleepovers at the house of her choice to support the transition and to experience the changes in routines. However, because she was moving from a family home into a supported tenancy, there were many differences, including how shopping was done, that jobs in the house were shared and having a different taxi driver to college. Some differences were due to service requirements, such as dispensing medication, finance checking and storing cleaning materials.

There was so much involved in moving house that not all of these differences could be explained in advance of the move. For months after the move, May's support staff continued to support her to understand the changes in her situation. This was achieved through very regular repetition, constant reassurance that it was okay that other people did things differently, using stories around specific issues, and a lot of work developing strategies for staff to support her to manage anxiety.

When Lauren's Mum died after a very rapid deterioration from apparently good health, Lauren appeared to cope with the loss very well, especially considering how close she was to her Mum. She attended the funeral and her Dad and sisters spent even more time with her to support her. Lauren carried around photographs of her Mum to prompt people to talk about her. However, several months later, Lauren's behaviour deteriorated. She began to hit out at her Dad, the other women she lived with, her friends at the day service and her support staff. She became more fixed in her routines, especially around food and clothing, and quickly became very agitated. She also became anxious around her age and when she might die. Lauren's Dad and her support staff felt that she was now experiencing the consequences of the loss of her Mum and was, understandably, having difficulty in coming to terms with the changes and the new information that this involved.

Lauren was referred to a counsellor who specialised in working with people with learning disabilities. She was also supported to draw pictures of her Mum, including the time she was in hospital and the funeral; to put flowers on the grave; to collect objects to remind her of her Mum and put them in a memory box, and to make a photo collage for her bedroom. Staff also used stories to help Lauren understand about death and to help her talk about her experience. When Lauren showed photographs or items from her memory box to her support staff or family, they spent time looking at them with her and talking to her about her Mum. Over time, Lauren became more settled, more flexible with her routines and less agitated and aggressive. She still talked about her Mum and carried photos of her; however, this became less frequent and was done with fondness rather than anxiety.

Speechmark

# Part 3
# Structuring for communication

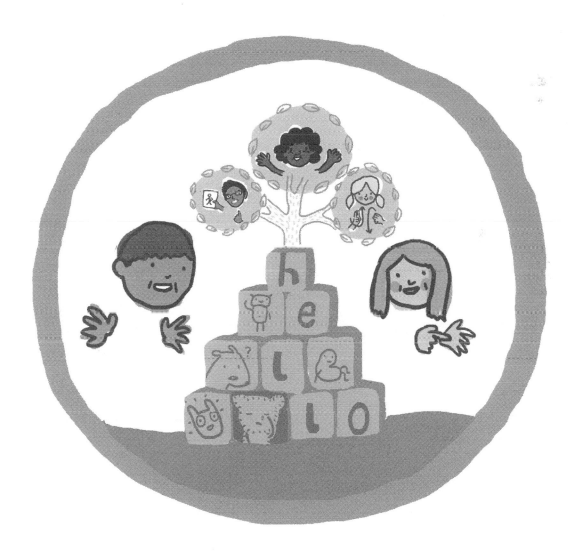

This part provides a set of steps to respond to the needs of people with a learning disability and create accessible environments.

# Making policies accessible

> **Policies are principles, rules, and guidelines formulated or adopted by an organization to reach its long-term goals. They are designed to influence and determine all major decisions and actions, and all activities take place within the boundaries set by them. Procedures are the specific methods employed to express policies in action in day-to-day operations of the organization. Together, policies and procedures ensure that a point of view held by the governing body of an organization is translated into steps that result in an outcome compatible with that view.**

(Business Dictionary.com, 2015)

Policies should reflect the ethos, values and work practice culture of a service; they are also a useful tool to guide the ethos, values and work practice culture of each employee. Policies can be used to influence change in work practice by giving structure and guidance to ensure consistency of work practice throughout a service. Policies are often based on legislation and best practice recommendations and they reflect the moral and ethical stance of how we should work with people with learning disabilities. Procedures within policies are used to inform daily practice. They should be written carefully, so that they do not restrict innovation, diversity and individual wishes or needs while protecting the people we support as well as the workforce.

The policies which directly affect people with a learning disability include:

- the complaints procedure

- equal opportunities and equality

- safeguarding

- bullying

- communication policy

- information and confidentiality.

Policies are generally written in concise and formal language. It is important to make policies accessible so that people with a learning disability can understand their rights and responsibilities and be safeguarded from malpractice. Making policies accessible to people with a learning disability is the first step towards empowering them to be involved in shaping the policies of the support and services that they access.

## Accessible complaints procedure

People have the right to complain about the services they use. However, it can be very difficult to access a complaints procedure, especially for people who do not use words to communicate. Enabling people to make a complaint or raise their concerns is important because it teaches them that they can say 'no' to something and express concerns over their care or the situations they are in.

It is not only barriers to communication that make it difficult to make a complaint. People may lack confidence, be wary of talking to people, have had bad experiences of making complaints in the past, or fear reprisal or further negative treatment if they do complain.

When writing the policy, consider the following issues.

- How the service raises awareness of how to make a complaint among the people it supports.

- Who can help a person make a complaint (eg a parent, a friend or an advocate).

- How to support someone to understand the process of the complaints procedure once a complaint is made. What will happen next and who will be involved?

- Accessible recording – make copies and/or feedback available for the person.

- Maintaining confidentiality.

- How to make people feel safe after making a complaint.

- How people supporting someone who doesn't communicate verbally can become aware of a complaints issue on their behalf from non-verbal methods of communication.

- How consent is gained to make a complaint on someone else's behalf, when this is needed and under which circumstances it may be a duty of care.

## Equal opportunities and equality

Understanding what equal opportunities are is part of upholding the rights of disabled people so that they have the opportunity to explore and challenge infringements.

When writing the policy, consider the following issues.

- What differences there are in society, eg disability, ethnicity, age, gender, sexuality, religion.

- What is understood by 'equal opportunities' and 'equality'.

- What is meant by 'fairness' and 'respect'.

- How the service promotes equal opportunities for its service users within the service and within the local community.

- What happens when people feel that they do not have equal opportunities or that there is not equality.

- Who can help a person take action.

- What the process would be.

- Accessible recording – make copies and/or feedback available for the person.

- How the service raises awareness of equal opportunities and equality among the people it supports.

## Safeguarding

People with a learning disability, particularly those who need support to communicate, form one of the most vulnerable groups in society. Wherever power relationships are unequal and people are supported in isolation, the opportunity for abuse is increased. Abuse can happen in any service. Safeguarding is about preventing this from occurring, or continuing, wherever possible; recognising and identifying abuse; ensuring that abuse is dealt with promptly and effectively, including notifying the appropriate agencies, including the police, where required. What many service policies omit is how to enable people to identify and report abuse themselves.

When writing the policy, consider the following issues.

- What is abuse? (eg financial, neglect, sexual, physical, psychological)

- What the service does to prevent abuse (eg checks on staff before they start the job, regular financial checks by managers).

- How people supporting someone who doesn't communicate verbally can become aware of abuse.

- Who can help someone talk about abuse (eg friend, family, staff, advocate).

- Supporting someone to communicate about abuse when they have limited or no verbal communication.

- Explaining the process once an issue is raised. What will happen next and who will be involved?

- How the service can support someone to cope more successfully with any unresolved issues after abuse.

- Maintaining confidentiality and protection.

- Accessible recording – making copies and/or feedback available for the person.

- How to make people feel safe after reporting abuse.

- How the service raises awareness of safeguarding issues among the people it supports.

## Bullying

Supporting people to understand that bullying is a form of abuse is an important part of safeguarding. This may form a separate policy or be part of the safeguarding policy. Talking about bullying can also make service users, as well as staff, aware of the impact that bullying can have on other people. It is important to recognise that service users can also bully other service users or members of staff.

When writing the policy, consider the following issues.

- What bullying is.

- Who can be bullied and who can be a bully.

- What it feels like to be bullied.

- How people who support a person who doesn't communicate verbally can become aware of bullying.

- Who can help someone talk about bullying (eg friend, family, staff, advocate).

- Supporting someone to communicate about bullying when they have limited or no verbal communication.

- Explaining the process once an issue is raised. What will happen next and who will be involved?

- Accessible recording – make copies and/or feedback available for the person.

- Maintaining confidentiality and protection.

**Speechmark**

- How to make people feel safe after reporting bullying.

- How the service raises awareness of safeguarding issues among the people it supports.

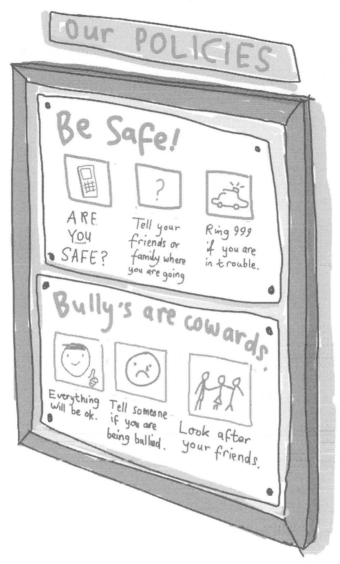

## Communication policy

The purpose of a communication policy is to set out the values and aims of a service around communication and making information accessible, to document how this should be achieved (with targets where work is in progress) and to outline the responsibilities of the people who work for the service.

When writing the policy, consider the following issues.

- What are the values of the service?

- What is the promise to service users around communication?

- How are these promises met?

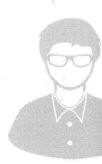

- Legislative/ or policy background

- An explanation regarding Total Communication and an outline of the methods used and promoted within the service.

- Guidelines around assessment, recording and reviewing of communication needs.

- Guidelines around making information accessible within the service.

- How people will be supported to communicate.

- Staff guidelines

- Resources and technology available within the service to support communication.

- Communication training made available to staff.

- Involvement of service users and families.

- Use of external support such as speech and language practitioners, experts on particular approaches.

- Funding allocation

- Quality assurance and the use of standardisation.

- Future aims for the service with targets.

## Information and confidentiality

All services hold information about the people they support. This information can enable the appropriate support to be offered and maintain people's safety. People have a right to know what information is kept about them and how this will be used or shared.

When writing the policy, consider the following issues.

- What information is held and why.

- Consent to keeping information.

- Where information is held.

- Who is allowed access to this information.

- What information might be shared, in what circumstances and with whom.

- People's right to see information that is kept about them.

- What confidentiality is.

- When confidentiality may be broken.

## Examples of good practice

A residential service for adults with a learning disability produces an accessible service user guide which includes a section on rights and responsibilities. This covers policies such as making a complaint, keeping safe, reporting abuse and equal opportunities. There is also a DVD which accompanies the accessible service user guide. Every year, staff and service users from the day service, which is run by the same organisation, produce an interactive play (for other service users) which explains what people's rights and responsibilities are.

A group of young people in a youth group which supports disabled and non-disabled young people has been given practical training in equality so that they can understand their rights and how to treat other people with respect. They learned about treating people fairly, about why some people are treated differently and how we can make things better for everyone. The young people helped to make a charter for young people's rights as a group and invited their local councillors to look at it.

A school for children with learning disabilities supported pupils to look at bullying by doing a project about it. This included making posters, role play and matching picture cards with emotion cards.

A group of young people were supported by an advocacy project to explore issues around safeguarding by creating a leaflet for other young people. Some of the subjects that were explored with the young people included times when they feel safe or unsafe, intimate care practice, things they would like to change, their right to whistle-blow and who they can talk to about any concerns.

A day service held a series of events around communication for people who accessed the service, their families and staff. At the end of the series, a consultation meeting took place between the service and those who accessed the service so that a charter on communication could be produced. The charter outlined what could be expected by people who attended the day service and how the service was to meet these expectations. This became the service's communication policy.

# Demonstrating elements underpinning continuing professional development

Continuing professional development (CPD) is essential to keeping work practice fresh. It is a great way of finding self-motivation and inspiration and reminds us of the purpose of our role and responsibilities to the people who we support. The best lessons that we learn are when we reflect on our daily practice by exploring what works, what does not work and new ways of doing things. In this way, we are constantly working towards improving our practice.

Sharing experiences with other people can support the development of our own and other practitioners' work practice and greatly contribute to changing or challenging the culture of the services we work in. Each practitioner can have a positive impact on the support that people receive and our own values can powerfully shape the daily experiences of the people we support. The process of CPD plays a vital role in enabling practitioners to check and further develop work practice.

All communication partners should be able to access CPD. Whether you work for a service specialising in supporting people with a learning disability, work for a community-based setting or organisation which includes people with a learning disability, are employed through direct payments, or are a family member or friend of someone with a learning disability, it is possible to access information, resources and support to develop your skills in communicating with and involving people.

Knowledge and skills can be developed through:

- training (eg structured, distance learning, work-based)
- self-reflection
- evaluation of personal and/or joint work practice
- mentoring or peer-mentoring
- coaching
- talking to people
- sharing practice and experiences
- observation
- structured discussion (eg through team meetings and action planning meetings)
- reading

- research on the internet
- visits to other workplaces or settings
- access to communication professionals such as speech and language therapists or a communication champion.

## Reflection

- Consider how you develop your work practice and skills. Which methods do you find are most beneficial?
- If applicable, how does your service support you to develop your skills and abilities in communicating with people who have learning disabilities?
- Consider how you could more actively take responsibility for developing your work practice.

## Personal continuing professional development

Learning new and developing existing skills in communication and involving people is a satisfying way of developing your practice. All individuals have a responsibility towards their continuing professional development. An individual who does not work within services may not have access to the resources, support and encouragement that others who work within a team or services have. Individual practitioners can develop their work practice incurring little expense, but this requires a more proactive and committed approach to professional development.

One of the most powerful ways of improving professional practice is by actively reflecting on how you work with people. This is most beneficial when done alongside reading or discussion with others which can challenge practitioners to analyse and develop work practice and evaluate what is done well.

Continuing professional development does not have to be done completely independently. Consider opportunities to improve your professional practice by visiting or shadowing a person at a place of work or joining an online forum or receiving online professional updates.

The structure of the *Communicate with Me* Quality Assurance Framework (see the online resource) has been designed to promote continuing professional work practice, ongoing reflection and sustainable changes to work practice for individual practitioners. The ultimate aim is to improve the quality of support that is offered to people with a learning disability.

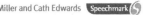

## Service-led continuing professional development

For many services, supporting teams to learn new skills and develop existing skills in communication and involving people will introduce a significant change in the way people work. The continuing professional development of practitioners promotes ongoing learning and the development of skills throughout an individual's career.

In addition to supporting practitioners to develop their knowledge and understanding, services need to nurture the transition from this to daily practice. The authors of *Communicate with Me* have observed that a major barrier to promoting positive change at the front line has not been the unwillingness of practitioners, nor the lack of individual skills, but the lack of resources and continued support to enable practitioners working at the front line, and their managers, to put what they have learned into practice.

Services may invest heavily in training; however, without the resources to support and develop newly acquired skills, the potential achieved through training may not be maximised. In fact, training can essentially become a tokenistic tick in a box for both practitioners and services if the knowledge and skills acquired through training are not transferred into work practice.

For example, a service trains some of its front-line practitioners to make information accessible to people with learning disabilities. This is a considerable resource commitment. Practitioners leave the training feeling enthusiastic, with new skills and new ideas about how they can support the people within their work setting more effectively. One month later, no changes are made and the training resources that were invested did not achieve their purpose. This was because of the following reasons.

- Individual practitioners were not working alongside team members who had received the same training, so practitioners were working on their own with no authority to promote new work practices within their team.

- Line managers had not received the training, so they were not aware of how to support change within the setting.

- No plan of action was made regarding how to introduce changes into work practice.

- Practitioners had no access to resources to make information accessible (such as a digital camera, a laminator or a computer and printer for symbols, pictures and photos).

- There was no access to further information, unless individuals sourced this themselves.

Speechmark

- There was no follow-up to monitor how practitioners were making progress.

- No one was available to provide further guidance and advice about putting into practice what was learned.

- Practitioners felt that they had no time to put into practice what they had learned.

- Motivation to make changes quickly diminished.

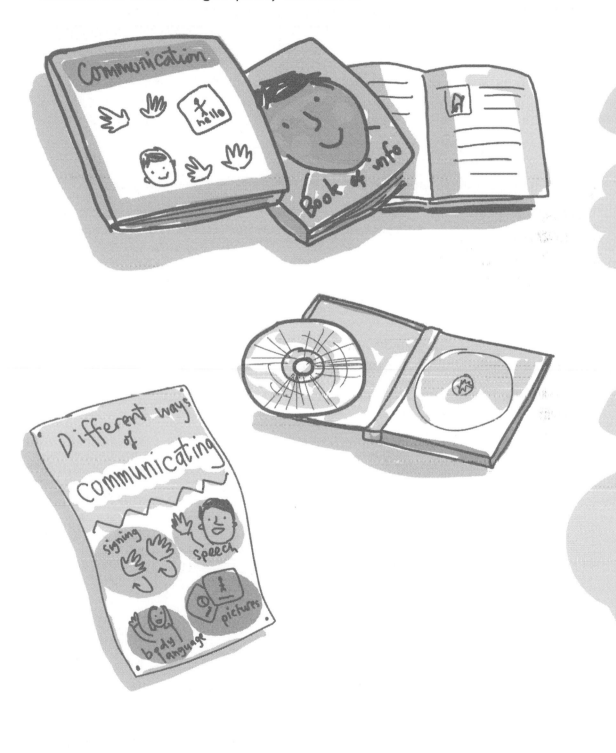

This section, along with the structure of *Communicate with Me* when used alongside the Quality Assurance Framework, supports managers to consider how to support teams to put into practice newly acquired skills and new ways of working. The ultimate aim of training (whether it is self-directed, or manager-led discussion within teams, or formal training) is to gain skills that can be put into practice to improve the support and opportunities offered to those who access the service.

To enable services and the individual practitioners they employ to achieve this aim, services need to provide the resources required, including:

- Resources and opportunities for practitioners to learn new skills.

- Resources and opportunities for practitioners to develop existing skills.

- Ongoing support from managers who also have the same skills and knowledge.

- Incentive to make changes by discussing and drawing up action plans within the team where individuals also have their own targets.

- Access to professionals for training, advice and guidance.

- Physical resources (eg for practitioners to make communication resources).

- Information and the means to access further information and do further research.

- Resources such as communication aids: for example, BIGmack™, electronic choice boards, a computer and software to enable practitioners to try what they have learned.

The structure of the *Communicate with Me* Quality Assurance Framework (see the online resource) has been designed to promote sustainable changes to work practice for individual practitioners, their teams and throughout services, with the ultimate aim of improving the quality of support that is offered to those who access our services.

## Examples of good practice

A supported tenancy network has started to build a collection of relevant articles, printed information from the internet and copied examples of good practice from within the service as a resource for practitioners. They have also made available a computer, digital camera, printer and laminator for practitioners to support people to make communication materials.

An afterschool play group for children with learning disabilities liaises with the schools that the children attend so that their play staff can learn from staff at the schools about how the children communicate and how best to support them.

Both the school and the afterschool play group recognise that the children and their staff benefit from this mutual exchange of information, so they have formalised the arrangement by organising joint training initiatives so that support, including communication and interaction, is consistent.

A youth group uses 'a sign a week' to support staff and other young people to use Makaton™ with each other. One young person with Down's syndrome is training to be a peer educator so that he can share his skills in Makaton with other young people and staff.

A day service employs a communication therapist for a day a week as their Communication Champion. He provides some in-house training around communication tools and work practices and meets with teams and individual practitioners to discuss specific issues around communication and involving people.

Managers at a short break setting added 'communication issues' to their fixed agenda in their team meetings and supervisions.

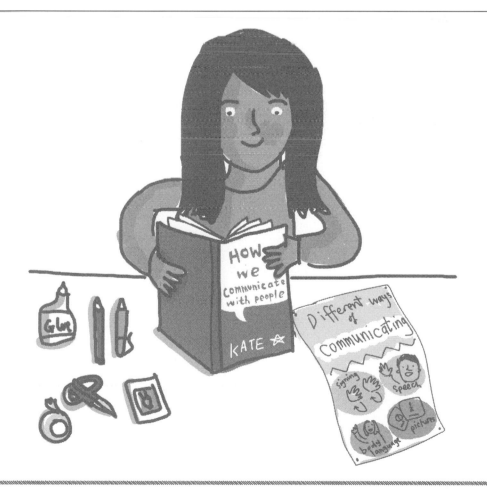

# References

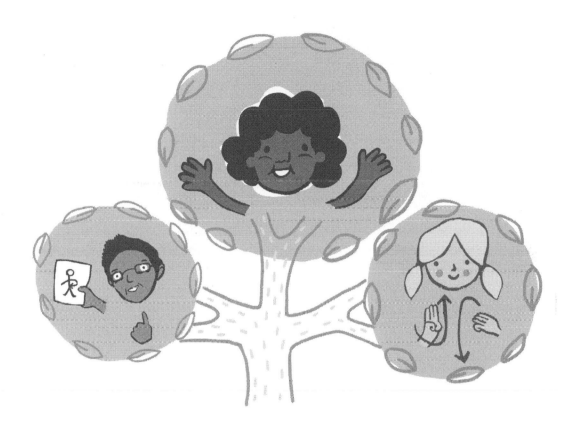

**Barbour A** (1976) *Louder than Words: Non-verbal Communication*, Merrill, Columbus, Ohio. Available online from: www.minoritycareernet.com.

**Barnes C** (1991) *Disabled People in Britain and Discrimination*, Hurst and Co., London.

**Brost M & Johnson T** (1982) *Getting to Know You – One Approach to Service Assessment and Planning for Individuals with Disabilities*, Wisconsin Council of Development Disabilities, Wisconsin.

**Business Dictionary.com** (2015) '*What are policies and procedures?*' (online), www.businessdictionary.com/definition/policies-and-procedures.html (accessed January 2015).

**Caldwell P & Horwood J** (2008) *Developmental Speech and Language Disorders*, Guilford Press, London.

**Caldwell P & Horwood J** (2008) *Using Intensive Interaction and Sensory Integration: a handbook for those who support people with severe autistic spectrum disorder*, Jessica Kingsley, London.

**Cantwell DP & Baker L** (1987) *Developmental Speech and Language Disorders*, Guilford Press, London.

**Child C** (2013) *Communication Development Profile*, Speechmark Publishing Ltd, Milton Keynes.

**Collis M & Lacey P** (1996) *Interactive Approaches to Teaching: A Framework for INSET*, David Fulton, London.

**Council of Europe** (2010) *European Convention on Human Rights* (online), www.echr.coe.int (accessed April 2015).

**Disability Discrimination Act** (1995, 2005), The Stationery Office, London.

**Disability Equality Duty** (2006), The Stationery Office, London.

**Equality Act** (2010), The Stationery Office, London.

**Finkelstein V** (1980) *Attitudes and Disabled People*. World Rehabilitation Fund, New York.

**Finkelstein V** (1981) 'To deny or not to deny disability', Brechin A *et al* (eds), *Handicap in a Social World*, Hodder and Stoughton, Sevenoaks.

**Goodwin M & Edwards C** (2009) 'I'm creative too', *PMLD Link*, 21 (1), pp11–17.

**Grove N** (2009) *Learning to Tell: a handbook for inclusive storytelling*, BILD, Kidderminster.

**Grove N** (2012) *Using Storytelling to Support Children and Adults with Special Needs: Transforming Lives Through Telling Tales*, David Fulton, London.

**Grove N** (2014) *The Big Book of Story Sharing*, Speechmark, London.

**Grove N & Park K** (2001) *Social Cognition through Drama and Literature*, Jessica Kingsley, London.

**Hansen B** (1980) *Aspects of Deafness and Total Communication in Denmark*, The Centre for Total Communication, Copenhagen.

**Human Rights Act** (1998) The Stationery Office, London.

**Jordan R** (1999) *Autistic Spectrum Disorders: an introductory handbook for practitioners*, David Fulton, Oxon.

**Kumin L** (2012) *Early Communication Skills for Children with Down Syndrome – A Guide for Parents and Professionals*, Woodbine House, Bethesda.

**Mansell J & Brown H** (2012) *Active Support – Enabling and Empowering People with Intellectual Disabilities*, Jessica Kingsley Publishers, London.

**Martin D** (2000) *Teaching Children with Speech and Language Difficulties*, David Fulton, London.

**Mencap** (2011) *Involve Me – Independent Evaluation Report,* Mencap/Foundation for People with Learning Disabilities, London.

**Mental Capacity Act** (2005), The Stationery Office, London.

**Money D & Thurman S** (1994) 'Talk about communication', *Bulletin of the College of Speech and Language Therapists*, 504, pp12–13.

**Nind M & Hewett D** (2005) *Access to Communication*, 2nd edn, David Fulton Publishers, London.

**O'Brien J & O'Brien L** (1981) *A Little Book About Person Centered Planning*, Inclusion Press, Toronto.

**O'Brien J, Pearpoint, J & Kahn L** (2010) *The PATH & MAPS Handbook: Person-Centered Ways to Build Community*, Inclusion Press, Toronto.

**Oliver M** (1990) *The Politics of Disablement*, Macmillan, Basingstoke.

**Oliver M** (1996) *Understanding Disability: From Theory to Practice*, Macmillan, Basingstoke.

**Puddephatt A** (2005) *Freedom of Expression – The Essentials of Human Rights*, Hodder Arnold, London.

**Reiser R & Mason M** (1990) *Disability Equality in the Classroom: A Human Rights Issue*, ILEA, London.

**Rowland C** (1996) *Communication Matrix*, Oregon Health Sciences University, Portland, Oregon.

**Sanderson H and Associates** (1997) *People, Plans and Possibilities: Exploring Person Centred Planning*, SHS Ltd, Edinburgh.

**Thurman S** (2011) 'Is communication a human right for people with profound and multiple learning disabilities?', *PMLD Link: Sharing Ideas and Information*, 23 (1), pp10–14.

**UN General Assembly** (1989) *Convention on the Rights of the Child*, United Nations, Treaty Series, vol. 1577, p3. Available online at: www.unhcr.org/refworld/docid/3ae6b38f0.html (accessed January 2012).

**UN General Assembly** (2006) *Convention on the Rights of Persons with Disabilities*, online, www.unhcr.org/refworld/docid/4680cd212.html (accessed January 2013).

**Voices through Advocacy** (VTA) (2008) *When Communication Gets Tough*, Scope, London.

**Ware J** (2004a) 'Ascertaining the views of people with profound and multiple learning disabilities', *British Journal of Learning Disabilities*, 32, pp175–9.

**Ware J** (2004b) *Creating a Responding Environment for People with Profound and Multiple Learning Difficulties*, David Fulton, London.

# Further reading and resources

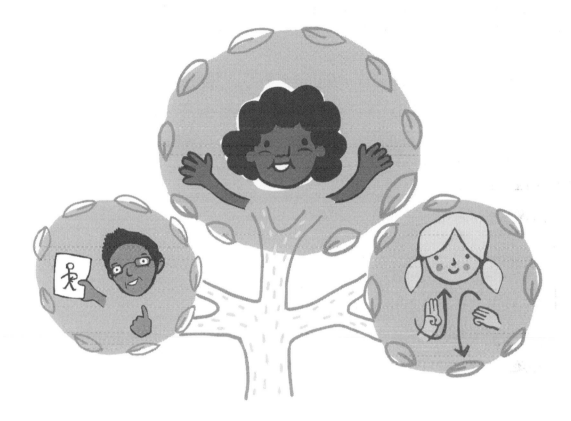

## Disability, the social and medical approaches

**Morris J** (1991) *Pride against Prejudice*, Women's Press, London.

**Oliver M** (1996) *Understanding Disability from Theory to Practice*, Macmillan Press, London.

**Shakespeare T** (1996) 'Disability, identity and difference', Barnes C & Mercer G (eds), *Exploring the Divide*, The Disability Press, Leeds.

**Shakespeare T** (2006) *Disability Rights and Wrongs*, Routledge, London.

## General communication with people with learning disability

**Fulton R & Richardson K** (2011) *Equality and Inclusion for Learning Disability Workers*, BILD, Kidderminster.

**Thurman S** (2009) *BILD Guide: Communication is a Human Right*, BILD, Kidderminster.

**Thurman S** (2011) *Communicating Effectively with People with a Learning Disability*, BILD, Kidderminster.

**Communication Matters** website: www.communicationmatters.org.uk

**National Autistic Society** website: www.nas.org.uk

**Royal College of Speech and Language Therapists** website: www.rcslt.org.uk

# Accessible websites

Making your website accessible for people with a learning disability: www.intrasolutions.co.uk/website accessibility.pdf

Using Widgit to make sites accessible: www.widgit.com/online/index.htm

W3C Quick Tips to make accessible websites: www.w3.org/WAI/quicktips

# Bereavement – resources to support communication

**Faherty C** (2008) *Understanding Death and Illness and What They Teach about Life: An Interactive Guide for Individuals with Autism or Aspergers and Their Loved Ones*, Future Horizons, Arlington, Texas.

A guide for professionals offering bereavement support: www.bereavementanddisability.org.uk/BSLD3.htm

Supporting people with autism to understand death (includes a further list of resources): www.ukautism.org/pdf/compass/understandingdeath.pdf

## Choice

**Department of Health** (2015) *Consent: a guide for people with learning disability*, online, www.dh.gov.uk/prod_consum_dh/groups/dh_digitalassets/@dh/@en/documents/digitalasset/dh_4019159.pdf

**Jackson E & Jackson N** (2002) *Helping People with a Learning Disability Explore Choice*, Jessica Kingsley Publishers, London.

**Thurman S** (no date) *BILD Guide: Making complaints work for people with learning disabilities*, BILD, Kidderminster.

## Communication with people who have more complex needs

**Grove N** (2000) *See What I Mean: Guidelines to aid understanding of communication by people with severe and profound learning disabilities*, BILD, Kidderminster.

**Bag Books**: www.bagbooks.org

**Communication and People with Complex Needs Guidance**: www.mencap.org.uk/page.asp?id=1539

**Fact sheets on assessing and developing pre-symbolic communication**: http://itcnew.idahotc.com/dnn/IdahoTrainingInitiatives/VideoFactSheetIntro/tabid/919/Default.aspx

**Mencap** guide to communicating with people with PMLD: www.mencap.org.uk/guides.asp?id=459

**Multimedia profiling**: www.acting-up.org.uk

**PMLD and art**: www.mencap.org.uk/guides.asp?id=322

## Documenting communication

**Sanderson H and Associates** (1997) *People, Plans and Possibilities: Exploring Person Centred Planning*, SHS Ltd, Edinburgh.

**Communication Dictionaries**: www.helensandersonassociates.co.uk/reading-room/how/person-centred-thinking/person-centred-thinking-tools/communication-charts.aspx

**Communication Passports**: www.communicationpassports.org.uk

## Exploring situations through storytelling

**Alexander J** (2004) *Going Up!: The No-Worries Guide to Secondary School*, A & C Black Publishers, London.

**Auld M** (2010) *Going on Holiday (My Family and Me)*, Franklin Watts, London.

**Hunter R** (2004) *Moving House*, Evans Publishing Group, London.

**Bag Books**: www.bagbooks.org

**Carol Gray**: resources and publications on a specific approach to storytelling: www.thegraycenter.org

**Downloadable story builder**: www.leedsmet.ac.uk/inn/usabilityservices/download2.htm

- Some free resources and material for purchase which can be individualised. Includes social situations such as 'school rules', 'bus rules', 'going to the doctor', 'getting along with people', 'bullying': www.sandbox-learning.com

- Some examples of social stories: www.polyxo.com/socialstories, http://kidscandream.webs.com/page12.htm

- Social story resources for teenagers with Asperger's covering teenage situations: www.autismsocialstories.com/asperger_adolescents

- Widgit downloads for social stories: www.widgit.com/resources/stories/teenagers/index.htm

## Interactive approaches

**Caldwell P** (2006) *Finding You Finding Me: Using Intensive Interaction to Get in Touch with People Whose Severe Learning Disabilities Are Combined with Autistic Spectrum Disorder*, Jessica Kingsley Publishers, London.

**Caldwell P** (2007) *From Isolation to Intimacy: Making Friends Without Words*, Jessica Kingsley Publishers, London.

**Kellett M & Nind M** (2003) *Implementing Intensive Interaction in Schools – Guidance for Practitioners, Managers and Coordinators*, David Fulton Publishers, London.

**Nind M** (1996) *Access to Communication: developing the basics of communication with people with severe learning disabilities through intensive interaction*, David Fulton, London.

**Nind M & Hewett D** (2001) *A Practical Guide to Intensive Interaction*, BILD, Kidderminster.

**Nind M & Hewett D** (2005) *Access to Communication*, 2nd edn, David Fulton, London.

**BILD** factsheet on Intensive Interaction – www.bild.org.uk/pdfs/05faqs/ii.pdf

**Dave Hewett** on Intensive Interaction: www.davehewett.com/intensive.php

**Phoebe Caldwell** on Intensive Interaction: www.phoebecaldwell.co.uk/work.html

## Legislation and policy

**Department for Education and Schools** (DfES) (2006) *Information Sharing: Practitioners' Guide*, DfES, London.

**Department for Education and Schools** (DfES) (2006) *Making It Happen: Working together for children, young people and families*, DfES, London. Available online at: www.everychildmatters.gov.uk/resources-and-practice/IG00130/.

**Disability Equality Duty**: www.dotheduty.org

**Mental Capacity Act** (simplified version): www.devon.gov.uk/contrast/mca-easy-summary.pdf

**Mental Capacity Act** (code of practice): http://webarchive.nationalarchives.gov.uk/ and www.dca.gov.uk/legal-policy/mental-capacity/mca-cp.pdf

**UN Convention on Disability Rights**: www.un.org/disabilities

## Making information accessible

**CHANGE:** www.changepeople.co.uk/uploaded/CHANGE_How_to_Make_Info_Accessible_guide.pdf

**Department of Health**: Making written information easier to understand for people with learning disabilities – Guidance for people who commission or produce 'easy read' information – revised edition 2010 (Section 4 includes guidance on how to involve people with learning disability): www.valuingpeoplenow.dh.gov.uk/webfm_send/377

**Thurman S, Jones J & Tarleton B** (2005) 'Without words – meaningful information for people with high individual communication needs', *British Journal of Learning Disabilities*, 33, pp83–89 (BILD publications). Available online at: www.bild.org.uk/humanrights/docs/seldom_heard/section_3/3_1/Resource_one_meaningful_information_article.pdf (accessed January 2015).

## Objects of reference

**Ockelford A** (2002) *Objects of Reference*, RNIB, London.

**Park K** (1997) 'How do objects become objects of reference? A review of the literature on objects of reference and a proposed model for the use of objects in communication', *British Journal of Special Education*, 24 (3), pp108–14.

**Park K** (2002) *Objects of Reference in Practice and Theory*, Sense, London.

**www.ace-centre.org.uk** (once on-site, search for 'objects of reference')

**www.rnib.org.uk** (once on-site, search for 'objects of reference')

**www.sense.org.uk** (once on-site, search for 'objects of reference')

## Person-centred planning

**O'Brien J & O'Brien CL** (1998) *A Little Book about Person Centered Planning*, Inclusion Press, Toronto.

**People First, Manchester and Liverpool** (1997) *Our Plan for Planning*, Manchester People First, Manchester.

**Sanderson H and Associates** (1997) *People, Plans and Possibilities: Exploring Person Centred Planning*, SHS Ltd, Edinburgh.

**British Institute of Learning Disability** information on person-centred planning: www.bild.org.uk/docs/05faqs/pcp.doc

**www.circlesnetwork.org.uk**

**www.disabilitydice.co.uk**

**www.helensandersonassociates.co.uk**

**www.inclusive-solutions.com**

## Signing

**British Sign Language**: www.british-sign.co.uk

**Deaf-blind signing**: www.deafblind.com

**Deaf-blind finger spelling translator**: www.deafsign.com (enter text and program translates it into sign)

**Makaton**: www.makaton.org

**Signalong**: www.signalong.org.uk

Things to take into consideration when supporting someone who is deaf-blind: www.deafblind.com/slmorgan.html

## Symbols

**Detheridge T & Detheridge M** (1997) *Literacy Through Symbols – Improving Access for Children and Adults*, David Fulton Publishers, London.

**Johnson M** (1995) *The Picture Communication Symbols Guide*, Mayer-Johnson Co., Pittsburgh, PA.

**ASD visual aids**: www.asdvisualaids.com

**Blissymbol**: www.blissymbols.co.uk, www.blissymbolics.org

**Makaton symbols**: www.makaton.org/about/about.htm

**PECS** (Picture Exchange Communication System), Pyramid Educational Consultants: www.pecs.org.uk, www.pecs.org.uk/general/what.htm; resources for communication tools: www.pecs.org.uk/shop/asp/default.asp

**Picture Communication Symbols**, Mayer-Johnson: www.mayer-johnson.com

**See Sense**: http://grids.sensorysoftware.com/Members/Sensory/see-sense-library

**Snaps photo bank**, Smartbox Assistive Technology: www.smartboxat.com/2011/02/snaps-photos-for-communication

**SymbolStix**: http://symbolstix.n2y.com/About.aspx

**Widgit**: www.widgit.com; www.widgit.com/symbols/index.htm#guides

## Technology

**Ace**: www.ace-centre.org.uk

**BIGmack**: www.bigmack.org

**Communication Matters**: www.communicationmatters.org.uk

**Find a Voice**: www.findavoice.org.uk

**Go Talk**: www.inclusive.co.uk/communication_aids/.../index.shtml

**Inclusive Technology Ltd**: www.inclusive.co.uk

**Orac**: www.lancs.ac.uk/depts/mardis/products/orac.html

**Speech bubble**: www.speechbubble.org.uk

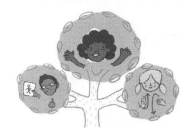

# What's next?

**Individuals can register to be part of the Communicate with Me – Communication Partner Development Scheme.**

- Be placed on the Communicate with Me – Communication Partner Development Scheme Register (viewable on the Communicate with Me website)*

- Receive Communicate with Me – Communication Partner Development Scheme Certificate for Individuals**

- Receive guidance to support the implementation of the Communication Partner Development Scheme

- Receive information on the future developments, additional materials and news of updates to quality assurance materials

**Services can register to be part of the Internal Quality Assurance Scheme for Services.**

- Be placed on the Communicate with Me – Internal Quality Assurance Scheme Register (viewable on the Communicate with Me website)*

- Receive the Communicate with Me Internal Quality Assurance Scheme Certificate for Services**

- Receive guidance to support the implementation of the Internal Quality Assurance Scheme for Services

- Receive information on the future developments, additional materials and news of updates to quality assurance materials

Register today

## www.communicatewithme.com

*Terms and conditions apply (see website).

**Additional payment required for the supply of certificates.